The Ped
Acute C
Handboo

The Pediatric Acute Care Handbook

Edited by

Mary Lieh-Lai, M.D.
Chief, Pediatric Intensive Care,
Children's Hospital of Michigan, Detroit

Maria Asi-Bautista, M.D.
Fellow in Critical Care Medicine,
Children's Hospital of Michigan/
Wayne State University School of Medicine

Katherine Ling-McGeorge, M.D.
Assistant Professor, Ambulatory Pediatrics,
Children's Hospital of Michigan/
Wayne State University School of Medicine

Little, Brown and Company
Boston   New York   Toronto   London

Library of Congress Cataloging-in-Publication Data

The pediatric acute care handbook / [edited by] Mary Liah-Lai.
    p.   cm.
  Includes bibliographical references and index.
  ISBN 0-316-09306-8
  1. Pediatric emergencies--Handbooks, manuals, etc. 2. Pediatric intensive care--Handbooks, manuals, etc.   I. Lieh-Lai, Mary.
  [DNLM: 1. Acute Disease--in infancy & childhood —handbooks.
  2. Critical Care—in infancy & childhood—handbooks. WS 39 P3701 1995]
  RJ370.P38 1995
  618.92'0025—dc20
  DNLM/DLC   95-9591
  for Library of Congress   CIP

Printed in the United States of America

RRD-VA

Notice.   Although great care has been taken in compiling and editing the information presented in this manual to ensure accuracy and thoroughness, neither the contributors nor Children's Hospital of Michigan can accept any responsibility for any errors or omissions, whether caused by negligence or otherwise, or any consequences whatsoever arising from the use of information contained in this manual.

Editorial: Nancy E. Chorpenning
Production Services: Editorial Services of New England
Cover Illustration: Lauren Heidemann, age 8
Second Printing

To Our Teacher, Sheldon Brenner, D.O. (1940–1993)

A university consists, and has ever consisted, in demand and supply in wants which it alone can satisfy and which it does satisfy, in the communication of knowledge, and the relation and bond which exist between the teacher and the taught.
—John Henry Newman

It is a privilege and an honor to be asked by Dr. Brenner's students to dedicate to him this handbook, which they prepared with the kind of commitment, discipline, and perseverance that would make Dr. Brenner proud. Dr. Brenner's association with Children's Hospital of Michigan was multifaceted. He was an intern, a resident, an attending physician, the chief of ambulatory pediatrics, the residency program director, and the chief of staff. I knew Sheldon for almost a quarter century. He taught me, and he learned from me. I laughed with him, and I fought with him. I praised him, and at times I criticized him. I worked with him mostly as an associate but occasionally even as an adversary. Regardless of one's relationship with Sheldon, one always came away with a deep sense of respect for this man of great integrity and dignity. He asked nothing of others that he would not ask of himself. I am certain that Dr. Brenner would have looked at his students' efforts leading to this handbook with a great deal of pride and satisfaction.

Dr. Brenner was truly inspirational to all of us during his valiant fight against his illness. He worked tirelessly until the very end, never quitting, and always giving. Death need not be proud, for it never came close to touching his spirit. His indomitable will and dedication remain with those whose lives he touched and will live forever.

Ashok P. Sarnaik, M.D.
Chief, Critical Care Medicine
Professor of Pediatrics
Children's Hospital of Michigan
Wayne State University School of Medicine

Contents

Contributors

Maria Asi-Bautista

Silvia Operti-Considine

Jolene Ellis

Paul Hennis

Frederick Klingbeil

Joan Less

Mary Lieh-Lai

Katherine Ling-McGeorge

Kushal Vinod Raghubir

Alexandre Rotta

Michelle Rotta

Sunita Sarin

Preface

The Pediatric Acute Care Handbook is based on the Critical Care Resident Educational Series (CCRES), which was conceived in 1991 as a bimonthly lecture series at Children's Hospital of Michigan. The lectures were organized for and by the pediatric house staff under the guidance of Dr. Mary Lieh-Lai, Director of the Intensive Care Unit.

The goal of CCRES is to prevent and decrease morbidity and mortality associated with acute life-threatening illnesses, injuries, or complications by enhancing the residents' appreciation and capabilities of identifying, investigating, treating, and monitoring these medical and surgical problems. CCRES was a response to the increasing acuity of patients facing today's health care system and the need for the physician *to provide more acute care management* outside *the intensive care unit*.

The series was highly successful, both in terms of resident participation and resident education. This handbook stems from that same commitment by the house staff at Children's Hospital of Michigan to continue their efforts to help provide good care to all sick children.

MLL
MAB
KLM

Acknowledgments

We wish to extend our sincerest gratitude to the following people who made this project possible:

The 1993 graduates of the pediatric residency program: Michael Anderson, MD; Brian Engel, MD; Maya Heinert, MD; and Frederick Klingbeil, MD, who came up with the idea of an educational series (CCRES), on which this handbook is based.

Curt Ellis and Katherine Ling-McGeorge, MD, for the illustrations used in the procedures section.

Faculty reviewers: Bassam Atiyeh, MD, Hyponatremia, Hypernatremia, HUS; Indira Warrier, MD, DIC, Hemophilia Emergencies; Shermine Dabbagh, MD, Acute Renal Failure, HUS; Peter Karpawich, MD, Dysrhythmias, EKG rhythm strips and commentaries; Sandra Clapp, MD, Dysrhythmias; Zia Farooki, MD, Congestive Heart Failure, Cyanotic Infant; Division of Endocrinology, Adrenal Crisis, Diabetic Protocol; James Cisek, MD, Toxicology; Suzanne White, MD, Toxicology; Sharada Sarnaik, MD, Sickle Cell Disease; Yaddanapudi Ravindranath, MD, Anemia; Ellen Moore, MD, HIV; Erawati Bawle, MD, Hyperammonemia; Division of Infectious Disease, Antibiotic Formulary; Diana Farmer, MD, Trauma; and especially Ashok Sarnaik, MD, for his time and patience in reviewing each topic and for his invaluable suggestions and criticisms.

Ed and Chris Lai, for putting up with us during our long brainstorming sessions in their home.

The second and third year residents (1993-1994) at Children's Hospital of Michigan for their comments and suggestions during the "trial run."

Guidelines for Use

This handbook was developed to help house officers in the initial stabilization and management of problems commonly encountered in the care of pediatric patients.

Algorithms begin with presenting signs and symptoms and the minimum workup required at the time of presentation.

(A) refers to annotations on the facing page.

☆ denotes a critical point, explained below the algorithm.

✱ indicates a continuing page.

☎_____ is a suggestion that the reader call for assistance with space provided for the reader to fill in appropriate phone numbers.

"Call Senior Resident" means to notify the senior pediatrician at the institution.

The aim of this handbook is to help house officers anticipate life-threatening complications, recognize when to call appropriate services, and transfer patients to a tertiary care center when these services are not available at their institution.

STAT doses are provided when necessary. The reader is encouraged to refer to standard text for details.

This handbook does not attempt to provide an exhaustive listing of differential diagnoses, and it should not be considered a substitute for recommended textbooks. A suggested reading list follows the text.

Management protocols were patterned after guidelines in use at Children's Hospital of Michigan. Other modalities are mentioned, but the reader should discuss these options with appropriate attending physicians.

Patients need to be reassessed frequently, and management must be tailored according to the patient's condition.

CCRES Rules

1. Know your ABCs: airway, breathing, circulation.
2. If you do not suspect, you do not diagnose.
3. Man scan (physical exam) is better than CAT scan.
4. In monitoring patients, know what to look for; know the benefits and limitations of monitoring.
5. ASSESS FREQUENTLY.
6. When unsure, always call for help. ☎
7. Patients can deteriorate very rapidly; act now!

List of Abbreviations

A

ABCs	airway, breathing, circulation
ABG	arterial blood gas
ACh	acetylcholine
AChe	acetylcholinesterose
ACD	acid citrate dextrose
ACTH	adrenocorticotropic hormone
ADH	antidiuretic hormone
AFB	acid fast bacilli
$Al(OH)_3$	aluminum hydroxide
ALT	alanine transferase
ALTE	apparent life-threatening event
AML	acute myelogenous leukemia
ANA	antinuclear antibody
ANC	absolute neutrophil count
AP	anterior posterior
ASAP	as soon as possible
ASD	atrial septal defect
ASO	antistreptolysin O
AST	aspartate transferase
ATN	acute tubular necrosis
ATP	adenosine triphosphate
A FIB	atrial fibrillation
AV	arteriovenous, atrioventricular
AVN	AV node
AVP	arginine vasopressin

B

BAL	bronchoalveolar lavage
BBB	bundle branch block
BID	twice a day
BMT	bone marrow transplant
BSA	body surface area
BSAB	body surface area burned
BP	blood pressure
BPD	bronchopulmonary dysplasia
bpm	beats per minute
BUN	blood urea nitrogen

C

C	centigrade
Ca^{+2}	calcium
CaCl	calcium chloride
$CaCO_3$	calcium carbonate
cap	capsule
$CaPO_4$	calcium phosphate
CBC	complete blood count
CBG	capillary blood gas
CF	cystic fibrosis

CHD	congenital heart disease
ChE	cholinesterase
CHF	congestive heart failure
CIE	counter immunoelectrophoresis
CN	cranial nerves
CNS	central nervous system
CO	cardiac output, carbon monoxide
coagulation profile:	PT, PTT, TT, FSP
COHb	carboxyhemoglobin
CO_2	carbon dioxide
CPK	creatine phosphokinase
CPR	cardiopulmonary resuscitation
CR monitor	cardiorespiratory monitor
CSF	cerebrospinal fluid
CT	computerized axial tomography
CVA	cerebrovascular accident
CVC	central venous catheter
CVP	central venous pressure
CVS	cardiovascular system

D

D	dextrose
D_5W	dextrose with water
DBP	diastolic blood pressure
DFO	deferoxamine
DI	diabetes insipidus
DIC	disseminated intravascular coagulation
div.	divided
DKA	diabetic ketoacidosis
dL	deciliter
DVT	deep vein thrombosis
DPL	diagnostic peritoneal lavage

E

ECF	extracellular fluid
ECMO	extracorporeal membrane oxygenation
EDTA	ethylenediaminetetraacetic acid
EEG	electroencephalogram
EKG	electrocardiogram
ELISA	enzyme linked immunosorbent assay
EMD	electromechanical dissociation
EMG	electromyogram
ENT	otorhinolaryngology
ESR	erythrocyte sedimentation rate
ET	endotracheal
EXT	extremities

F

Fe	iron
FE_{Na}	fractional excretion of sodium
FEV_1	forced expiratory volume in 1 second
FFP	fresh frozen plasma

FIB	fibrillation
FiO$_2$	fraction of inspired oxygen
FSP	fibrin split products
FTT	failure to thrive
FVC	forced vital capacity

G

g	gram
GBS	Guillain-Barré syndrome
GCS	Glasgow Coma Scale
GI	gastrointestinal
GPI	glucose phosphate isomerase
GU	genitourinary
G6PD	glucose-6-phosphate dehydrogenase

H

H$^+$	hydrogen ion
Hb	hemoglobin
HbSC	hemoglobin SC
HbSS	hemoglobin SS
HCG	human chorionic gonadotropin
HCO$_3$	bicarbonate
Hct	hematocrit
HEENT	head, eyes, ears, nose, throat
HEME	hematology
HeliOx	helium oxygen
HIV	human immunodeficiency virus
hr	hours
hpf	high power field
HTN	hypertension
HR	heart rate
HUS	hemolytic uremic syndrome

I

ICF	intracellular fluid
ICP	intracranial pressure
ICU	intensive care unit
IHSS	idiopathic hypertrophic subaortic stenosis
IM	intramuscular
INH	isoniazid
IO	intraosseous
I's and O's	input and output
IV	intravenous

J

J	Joules
JRA	juvenile rheumatoid arthritis
JVD	jugular venous distension

K

| K | potassium |

kg	kilogram
K_2PO_4	potassium phosphate
KCl	potassium chloride

L

L	liter
LDH	lactic dehydrogenase
LFT	liver function test
LIP	lymphocytic interstitial pneumonitis
LLQ	left lower quadrant
LMP	last menstrual period
LOC	loss of, or level of, consciousness
LP	lumbar puncture
LR	lactated Ringer's solution
LSD	lysergic acid diethylanude
LUQ	left upper quadrant
LVOTO	left ventricular outflow tract obstruction

M

MAP	mean arterial pressure
MCV	mean corpuscular volume
mEq/kg	milliequivalent per kilogram
mEq/L	milliequivalent per liter
max.	maximum
Mg^{+2}	magnesium
mg	milligram
MG	myasthenia gravis
mg	microgram
min	minutes
min.	minimum
ml	milliliter
mmHg	millimeters of mercury
mos	months
mOsm/L	milliosmoles per liter
MRI	magnetic resonance imaging

N

N	normal
Na^+	sodium
NaCl	sodium chloride
$NaHCO_3$	sodium bicarbonate
NaOH	sodium hydroxide
NEC	necrotizing enterocolitis
NG	nasogastric
NGT	nasogastric tube
NH_3	ammonia
NICU	neonatal intensive care unit
NPO	nothing by mouth
NS	normal saline
NSAID	nonsteroidal antiinflammatory drug

O

O_2	oxygen
OR	operating room

P

P	phosphorus
PA	pulmonary atresia, pulmonary artery
PAC	premature atrial complex
$PaCO_2$	partial pressure of CO_2
PAN	polyarteritis nodosa
PaO_2	partial pressure of O_2
PAT	paroxysmal atrial tachycardia
PCA	patient-controlled analgesia
PCC	prothrombin complex concentrate
PCP	pneumocystis carinii pneumonia
PDA	patent ductus arteriosus
PEA	pulseless electrical activity
PEFR	peak expiratory flow rate
PGE_1	prostaglandin E_1
PID	pelvic inflammatory disease
PK	pyruvate kinase
PLEDS	paroxysmal lateralizing epileptiform discharges
PMN	polymorphonuclear
PO	by mouth
PPD	purified protein derivative
PPHN	persistent pulmonary hypertension of the newborn
PR	per rectum
prn	as needed
PRBC	packed red blood cells
PT	prothrombin time
PTS	pediatric trauma score
PTT	partial thromboplastin time
PVC	premature ventricular complex
PVR	pulmonary vascular resistance
PEEP	positive end expiratory pressure

Q

q	every
QID	four times a day
QT_c	corrected QT interval

R

RBC	red blood cell
RDS	respiratory distress syndrome
RESP	respiratory
RDW	red cell distribution width
RLQ	right lower quadrant
RSV	respiratory syncytial virus
RR	respiratory rate
RTA	renal tubular acidosis
RUQ	right upper quadrant
RV	right ventricle
RVOT	right ventricular outflow tract

S

SBP	systolic blood pressure
Sßthal	sickle-beta thalassemia
SC	subcutaneous
SCI	spinal cord injury
SCID	severe combined immunodeficiency
sec	seconds
SGOT	serum glutamic oxalotransferase
SGPT	serum glutamic pyruvate transferase
SI	serum iron
SIADH	syndrome of inappropriate antidiuretic hormone secretion
Sinus tach	sinus tachycardia
SIRS	systemic inflammatory response syndrome
SL	sublingual
SLE	systemic lupus erythematosus
SPAG	small particle aerosol generator
STAT	at once
SV	stroke volume
SVR	systemic vascular resistance
SVT	supraventricular tachycardia

T

TB	tuberculosis
TBW	total body water
^{99}Tc-DMSA	technetium 99m-labeled dimercaptosuccinic acid
TDD	total digitalizing dose
THAM	tris-hydroxy-methyl-amino-methane
TIA	transient ischemic attack
TIBC	total iron binding capacity
TID	three times a day
TMP/SMZ	trimethoprim-sulfamethoxazole
TPN	total parenteral nutrition
TT	thrombin time
TTP	thrombotic thrombocytopenic purpura

U

U	unit
UAC	umbilical artery catheter
U_{Na}	urine sodium
URI	upper respiratory tract infection
US	ultrasound
UTI	urinary tract infection
UUN	urine urea nitrogen
UVC	umbilical vein catheter

V

VCUG	voiding cystourethrogram
Vd	volume of distribution
V FIB	ventricular fibrillation
VP	ventriculoperitoneal
V/Q	ventilation/perfusion

| VSD | ventricular septal defect |
| V tach | ventricular tachycardia |

W

| WBC | white blood cell |
| WPW | Wolff-Parkinson-White syndrome |

Y

| yr | years |

Notice.

The indications and dosages of all drugs in this book have been recommended in the medical literature and conform to the practices of the general medical community. The medications described do not necessarily have specific approval by the Food and Drug Administration for use in the diseases and dosages for which they are recommended. The package insert for each drug should be consulted for use and dosage as approved by the FDA. Because standards for usage change, it is advisable to keep abreast of revised recommendations, particularly those concerning new drugs.

ABCs/CPR

1 ABCs

- ABCs
- Cardiopulmonary Resuscitation

ABCs

Mary Lieh-Lai

(A) Ensure that the bulb is attached securely to the blade. If using a cuffed tube, ascertain cuff integrity by inflating cuff with a 3-5 ml syringe. Deflate cuff before insertion. After intubating, auscultate; ascertain equality of air entry; tape tube at the correct level.

(B) **Assess**, always assess!
Listen for air entry.
Check: EKG
         pulses—especially after defibrillating
         bedside blood sugar
         chest radiograph for ET placement.
Measure blood gases.

(C) **Access** is vital. Peripheral venous access should immediately be started; if unsuccessful after 2 attempts, proceed to IO needle placement (see p 205). Never defer these means of securing venous access while waiting for someone to perform a venous cutdown—this usually takes some time.

(D) **Breathing:** Use a properly fitted mask to ensure tight seal. Remember that not all patients who exhibit spontaneous respirations are able to maintain adequate ventilation/ oxygenation. If clinical signs and symptoms suggest overt respiratory failure, start bag and mask ventilation. Patients with ineffective breathing need ventilatory assistance before they develop apnea.

(E) **Drugs:** See p 229 for doses.

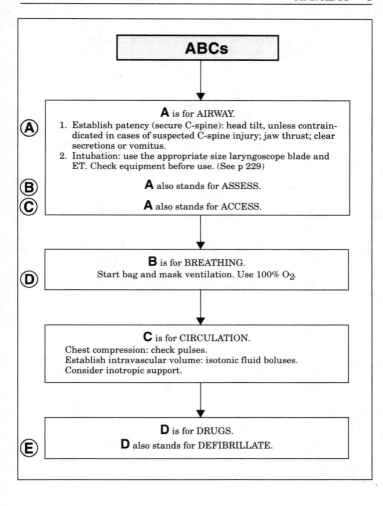

ABCs

(A) **A** is for AIRWAY.
1. Establish patency (secure C-spine): head tilt, unless contraindicated in cases of suspected C-spine injury; jaw thrust; clear secretions or vomitus.
2. Intubation: use the appropriate size laryngoscope blade and ET. Check equipment before use. (See p 229)

(B) **A** also stands for ASSESS.
(C) **A** also stands for ACCESS.

(D) **B** is for BREATHING.
Start bag and mask ventilation. Use 100% O$_2$.

C is for CIRCULATION.
Chest compression: check pulses.
Establish intravascular volume: isotonic fluid boluses.
Consider inotropic support.

(E) **D** is for DRUGS.
D also stands for DEFIBRILLATE.

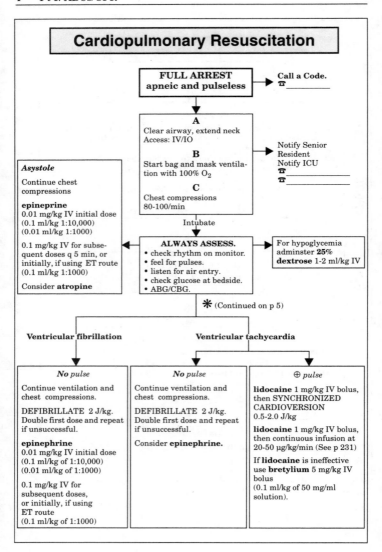

Cardiopulmonary Resuscitation

FULL ARREST
apneic and pulseless

Call a Code.
☎ _____

A
Clear airway, extend neck
Access: IV/IO

B
Start bag and mask ventilation with 100% O$_2$

C
Chest compressions
80-100/min

Notify Senior
Resident
Notify ICU
☎ _____
☎ _____

Intubate

ALWAYS ASSESS.
- check rhythm on monitor.
- feel for pulses.
- listen for air entry.
- check glucose at bedside.
- ABG/CBG.

For hypoglycemia
adminster **25%**
dextrose 1-2 ml/kg IV

Asystole

Continue chest
compressions

epineprine
0.01 mg/kg IV initial dose
(0.1 ml/kg 1:10,000)
(0.01 ml/kg 1:1000)

0.1 mg/kg IV for subsequent doses q 5 min, or
initially, if using ET route
(0.1 ml/kg 1:1000)

Consider **atropine**

✳ (Continued on p 5)

Ventricular fibrillation

Ventricular tachycardia

No pulse

Continue ventilation and
chest compressions.

DEFIBRILLATE 2 J/kg.
Double first dose and repeat
if unsuccessful.

epinephrine
0.01 mg/kg IV initial dose
(0.1 ml/kg of 1:10,000)
(0.01 ml/kg of 1:1000)

0.1 mg/kg IV for
subsequent doses,
or initially, if using
ET route
(0.1 ml/kg of 1:1000)

No pulse

Continue ventilation and
chest compressions.

DEFIBRILLATE 2 J/kg.
Double first dose and repeat
if unsuccessful.

Consider **epinephrine.**

⊕ *pulse*

lidocaine 1 mg/kg IV bolus,
then SYNCHRONIZED
CARDIOVERSION
0.5-2.0 J/kg

lidocaine 1 mg/kg IV bolus,
then continuous infusion at
20-50 µg/kg/min (See p 231)

If **lidocaine** is ineffective
use **bretylium** 5 mg/kg IV
bolus
(0.1 ml/kg of 50 mg/ml
solution).

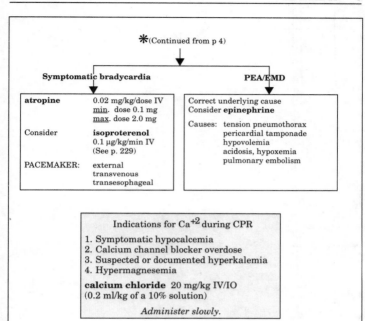

✱(Continued from p 4)

Symptomatic bradycardia

atropine	0.02 mg/kg/dose IV <u>min</u>. dose 0.1 mg <u>max</u>. dose 2.0 mg
Consider	**isoproterenol** 0.1 µg/kg/min IV (See p. 229)
PACEMAKER:	external transvenous transesophageal

PEA/EMD

Correct underlying cause
Consider **epinephrine**

Causes: tension pneumothorax
pericardial tamponade
hypovolemia
acidosis, hypoxemia
pulmonary embolism

Indications for Ca^{+2} during CPR

1. Symptomatic hypocalcemia
2. Calcium channel blocker overdose
3. Suspected or documented hyperkalemia
4. Hypermagnesemia

calcium chloride 20 mg/kg IV/IO
(0.2 ml/kg of a 10% solution)

Administer slowly.

Notes

Critical Conditions

2 Cardiovascular
- Congestive Heart Failure
- Cyanotic Infant
- Cardiac Dysrhythmias
- "Tet" Spells of Tetralogy of Fallot (TOF)
- Hypovolemic and Cardiogenic Shock

3 Child Abuse

4 Endocrine
- Adrenal Crisis
- Central Diabetes Insipidus
- Diabetic Ketoacidosis
- Syndrome of Inappropriate Antidiuretic Hormone Secretion

5 Gastrointestinal
- Acute Abdominal Pain
- Lower Gastrointestinal Bleeding
- Upper Gastrointestinal Bleeding

6 Hematology and Oncology
- Anemia
- Disseminated Intravascular Coagulation
- Hemophilia Emergencies
- Neutropenia with Fever
- Sickle Cell Disease
- Tumor Lysis Syndrome Hyperuricemia
- Tumor Lysis Syndrome Hyperphosphatemia (and Associated Hypocalcemia)

7   Immunology
- Anaphylaxis
- HIV ⊕ Patient with Fever
- HIV ⊕ Patient with Suspected Lung Involvement
- Acute Transfusion Reaction

8   Infectious Diseases
- Encephalitis
- Meningitis
- Septic Shock

9   Ingestions
- General Poisoning
- Acetaminophen Toxicity
- Alcohol Ingestions: Ethanol, Isopropanol, Methanol, Ethylene Glycol
- Caustic Ingestion/Exposure
- Cyclic Antidepressant Overdose
- Hydrocarbon Exposure
- Iron Poisoning
- Organophosphate/Carbamate Poisoning
- Theophylline Toxicity

10   Metabolic
- Acute Neonatal Hyperammonemia

11   Neurologic
- Coma
- Guillain-Barré Syndrome
- Increased Intracranial Pressure
- Myasthenia Gravis
- Spinal Cord Injury
- Status Epilepticus

12   Renal Fluids and Electrolytes

- Acute Renal Failure
- Hemolytic Uremic Syndrome
- Hypertensive Crisis
- Hypernatremia
- Hyponatremia
- Hyperkalemia
- Hypocalcemia
- Metabolic Acidosis

13   Respiratory

- Acute Bronchiolitis
- Acute Respiratory Failure
- Apnea
- Asthma
- Patient with Suspected Croup
- Dislodged Tracheostomy Tube
- Epiglottitis
- Foreign Body Aspiration

14   Smoke Inhalation and Surface Burns

- Burns: Thermal, Chemical, Electrical
- Smoke Inhalation Injury and Carbon Monoxide Poisoning

15   Trauma

- Stabilization of the Trauma Patient

Cardiovascular

Congestive Heart Failure

Paul Hennis and Katherine Ling-McGeorge

> - CHF represents a syndrome that results from the inability of the heart to provide adequate support for the metabolic requirements of the body. Symptoms are related to the failing heart and venous congestion. These include tachycardia, hepatomegaly, JVD. Clinicians must, however, be aware that extracardiac symptoms may be the primary manifestations of CHF, and these include respiratory distress (tachypnea and wheezing) and growth failure. CHF should be considered in children who present with frequent episodes of "pneumonia," tachypnea, or wheezing unresponsive to bronchodilators.
> - Cardiac Output (CO) = Heart Rate (HR) X Stroke Volume (SV).
> - Stroke volume is determined by three factors: preload, contractility, and afterload.

Etiologies of CHF

Pressure overload (obstructive and restrictive):
  pericardial effusion, LVOTO (coarctation of the aorta, aortic stenosis, interrupted aortic arch, hypoplastic left heart syndrome), systemic hypertension, pulmonary vascular obstructive disease

Volume overload:
  left-to-right shunts (PDA, VSD), valve regurgitation, severe anemia, systemic AV fistulae (liver, lung, brain)

Impaired myocardial function:
  cardiomyopathy, endo/myocarditis, ischemia (anomalous left coronary artery), dysrhythmia, endocardial fibroelastosis, toxins, drugs, hypoglycemia, storage disease

(A) If the child is known to have congenital heart disease or previous cardiac surgeries, review old chart. Determine doses of medications taken at home, including recent changes. Inquire about weight gain or lack of weight gain.

(B) If chronic airway obstruction with resultant cor pulmonale is suspected, inquire about URI, tonsillitis, snoring, somnolence.

(C) Occasionally, children may present with CHF secondary to cardiac tamponade. Causes include:

1. Pyogenic pericarditis: *Staphylococcus, Streptococcus, Neisseria meningitidis.* Staphylococcal pericarditis is sometimes observed following varicella infection.
2. Tuberculous pericarditis
3. Viral pericarditis
4. Tumors
5. Others: such as those associated with collagen vascular disease, SLE.

✳(Continued on p 12)

(A)
Clinical Manifestations

GENERAL failure to thrive, prolonged feeding, diaphoresis, cyanosis
CVS orthopnea, tachycardia, gallop rhythm, jugular venous distention, +/- murmur, +/- hyperdynamic precordium
RESP cough, dyspnea, wheezing, tachypnea
GI hepatomegaly
EXT +/- peripheral edema, poor peripheral pulses, pulsus alternans, cool extremities, prolonged capillary refill

Diagnostics

Blood ABG/CBG, CBC, differential, platelets, BUN, creatinine, electrolytes, Ca^{+2}, Mg^{+2}, glucose, lactic acid. Consider comprehensive drug screen, sepsis workup.
Urine urinalysis. Consider metabolic screen, comprehensive drug screen.
Others EKG, chest radiograph: cardiomegaly, Kerley's B lines, fluffy infiltrate

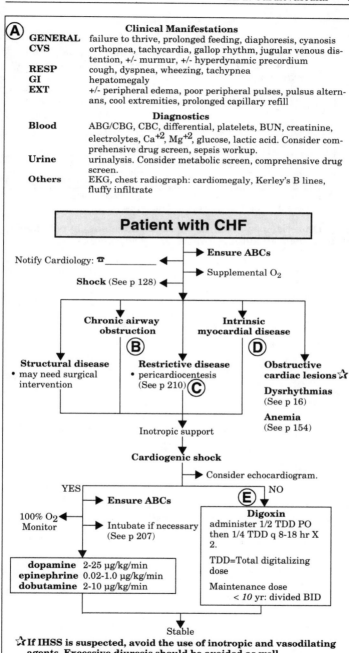

Patient with CHF

Notify Cardiology: ☎_____ ◄ ────► **Ensure ABCs**

────► Supplemental O_2

Shock (See p 128) ◄

Chronic airway obstruction
(B)

Intrinsic myocardial disease
(D)

Structural disease
• may need surgical intervention

Restrictive disease
• pericardiocentesis (See p 210) (C)

Obstructive cardiac lesions ☆

Dysrhythmias (See p 16)

Anemia (See p 154)

Inotropic support

Cardiogenic shock

────► Consider echocardiogram.

YES   NO

(E)

────► **Ensure ABCs**

100% O_2 ◄
Monitor

────► Intubate if necessary (See p 207)

Digoxin
administer 1/2 TDD PO then 1/4 TDD q 8-18 hr X 2.

TDD=Total digitalizing dose

Maintenance dose
< *10* yr: divided BID

dopamine 2-25 μg/kg/min
epinephrine 0.02-1.0 μg/kg/min
dobutamine 2-10 μg/kg/min

Stable

☆ **If IHSS is suspected, avoid the use of inotropic and vasodilating agents. Excessive diuresis should be avoided as well.**

✱(Continued on page 13)

✱(Continued from p 10)

(D)   Intrinsic myocardial disease: myocarditis (viral), vasculitis (Kawasaki's disease), ischemia (anomalous coronary
artery and hypoxia), storage diseases, muscular dystrophy

(E)   Digoxin dosing

Age	TDD in µg/kg/24 hr		Maintenance in µg/kg/24 hr	
	PO	IV/IM	PO	IV/IM
Premature	20	15	5	3-4
full-term	30	20	8-10	6-8
< 2 yr	40-50	30-40	10-12	7.5-9
2-10 yr	30-40	20-30	8-10	6-8
> 10 yr	750-1250		125-250	

Source: From Greene MG. *The Harriet Lane Handbook*, 1991, 12th ed, p
245. Mosby-Year Book, Inc, St Louis. With permission.

(F)   Diuretic use: monitor for hyponatremia, hypokalemia,
metabolic alkalosis, elevated uric acid, ototoxicity.

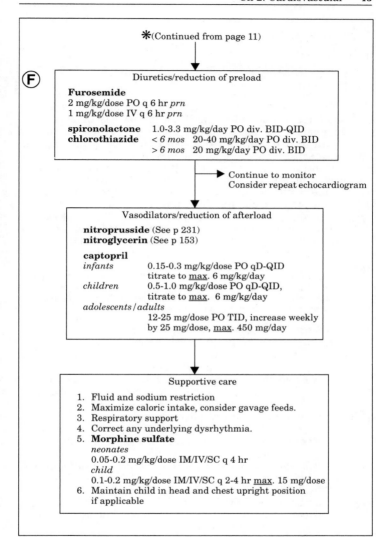

✴(Continued from page 11)

Ⓕ

Diuretics/reduction of preload

Furosemide
2 mg/kg/dose PO q 6 hr *prn*
1 mg/kg/dose IV q 6 hr *prn*

spironolactone		1.0-3.3 mg/kg/day PO div. BID-QID
chlorothiazide	*< 6 mos*	20-40 mg/kg/day PO div. BID
	> 6 mos	20 mg/kg/day PO div. BID

Continue to monitor
Consider repeat echocardiogram

Vasodilators/reduction of afterload

nitroprusside (See p 231)
nitroglycerin (See p 153)

captopril
infants   0.15-0.3 mg/kg/dose PO qD-QID
               titrate to <u>max</u>. 6 mg/kg/day
children   0.5-1.0 mg/kg/dose PO qD-QID,
               titrate to <u>max</u>. 6 mg/kg/day
adolescents / adults
               12-25 mg/dose PO TID, increase weekly
               by 25 mg/dose, <u>max</u>. 450 mg/day

Supportive care

1. Fluid and sodium restriction
2. Maximize caloric intake, consider gavage feeds.
3. Respiratory support
4. Correct any underlying dysrhythmia.
5. **Morphine sulfate**
    neonates
    0.05-0.2 mg/kg/dose IM/IV/SC q 4 hr
    child
    0.1-0.2 mg/kg/dose IM/IV/SC q 2-4 hr <u>max</u>. 15 mg/dose
6. Maintain child in head and chest upright position
    if applicable

Cyanotic Infant

Paul Hennis

> Cyanosis is defined as blue skin discoloration and is classified as either central or peripheral.

(A) In the presence of retractions, flaring, and grunting, consider respiratory etiology. If the patient is quiet and tachypneic, consider a cardiac etiology. A single S_2 may be heard in patients with transposition of the great arteries, tetralogy of Fallot, and pulmonary atresia.

(B) Central cyanosis: secondary to reduced hemoglobin in excess of 3 g/dL; more apparent with polycythemia, less with anemia. May be observed better in lips, mucous membranes, tongue, conjunctivae, nose tip.

(C) Peripheral cyanosis: secondary to (1) decreased cardiac output and subsequent decreased blood flow and increased O_2 peripheral extraction, (2) peripheral vasoconstriction.

(D)
> ### Hyperoxia test
>
> Administer 100% O_2 for 5-10 min. Obtain blood samples from the right radial or brachial artery (proximal to the patent ductus arteriosus), and analyze for PaO_2. Oxygen may cause closure of the ductus; monitor patient carefully during the procedure.

(E) Abnormal hemoglobin: methemoglobin, CO poisoning.
Respiratory etiology—V/Q mismatch:
- intrinsic   hypoventilation, airway obstruction, parenchymal disease
- extrinsic   diaphragmatic hernia, pneumothorax, pneumomediastinum, transient tachypnea of the newborn, RDS

(F) Characteristic chest radiograph findings
egg on a string: transposition of the great arteries
boot-shaped heart: tetralogy of Fallot/pulmonary atresia/VSD
snowman sign: supracardiac total anomalous pulmonary venous return
wall-to-wall heart: Ebstein's anomaly

(G) Characteristic EKG findings
superior left axis: tricuspid atresia, endocardial cushion defect, primum ASD
left axis deviation: pulmonary atresia, +/- tricuspid atresia
marked right atrial hypertrophy: Ebstein's anomaly

(H) Side effects of PGE_1: **apnea**, fever, flushing, tachy/bradycardia, **hypotension**, cardiac arrest. If patient worsens with PGE_1 infusion, consider total anomalous pulmonary venous return.

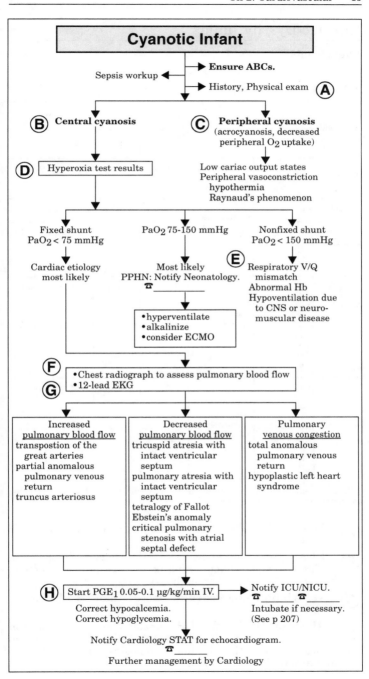

Cyanotic Infant

Sepsis workup ◄——— ▶ **Ensure ABCs.**
——▶ History, Physical exam **(A)**

(B) Central cyanosis   **(C) Peripheral cyanosis**
(acrocyanosis, decreased
peripheral O_2 uptake)

(D) Hyperoxia test results

Low cariac output states
Peripheral vasoconstriction
hypothermia
Raynaud's phenomenon

Fixed shunt PaO_2 75-150 mmHg   Nonfixed shunt
PaO_2 < 75 mmHg PaO_2 < 150 mmHg

Cardiac etiology   Most likely   **(E)** Respiratory V/Q
most likely   PPHN: Notify Neonatology.   mismatch
                        ☎_____   Abnormal Hb
                                                     Hypoventilation due
                                                     to CNS or neuro-
                        •hyperventilate   muscular disease
                        •alkalinize
                        •consider ECMO

(F) •Chest radiograph to assess pulmonary blood flow
(G) •12-lead EKG

Increased <u>pulmonary blood flow</u>	Decreased <u>pulmonary blood flow</u>	Pulmonary <u>venous congestion</u>
transpostion of the great arteries	tricuspid atresia with intact ventricular septum	total anomalous pulmonary venous return
partial anomalous pulmonary venous return	pulmonary atresia with intact ventricular septum	hypoplastic left heart syndrome
truncus arteriosus	tetralogy of Fallot Ebstein's anomaly critical pulmonary stenosis with atrial septal defect	

(H) Start PGE_1 0.05-0.1 µg/kg/min IV.   ——▶ Notify ICU/NICU.
                                                ☎_____ ☎_____
Correct hypocalcemia.   Intubate if necessary.
Correct hypoglycemia.   (See p 207)

Notify Cardiology STAT for echocardiogram.
☎_____
Further management by Cardiology

Cardiac Dysrhythmias

Paul Hennis

Table 2-1.

Dysrhythmia		Dose	Max. Initial Dose	Subsequent Doses	
				< 50 kg	> 50 kg
V FIB		Defibrillate 2 → 4 J/kg asynchronous	200 J	4 J/kg	200-300 J, 360 J
Atrial fibrillation*		Synchronized cardioversion 0.5 → 2 J/Kg	100 J	2 J/kg	200 J, 300 J, 360 J
Atrial flutter*			50 J		100 J, 200 J, 300 J, 360 J
SVT PAT					
⊖ pulse	V tach with regular form and rate	Defibrillate 2 → 4 J/kg asynchronous	100 J	4 J/kg	200 J, 300 J, 360 J
	V tach with *irregular* form and rate		200 J		200-300 J, 360 J
⊕ pulse	V tach with regular form and rate	Synchronized cardioversion 0.5 → 2 J/Kg	100 J	2 J/kg	200 J, 300 J, 360 J
	V tach with *irregular* form and rate		200 J		200-300 J, 360 J

* Following surgical correction, children with congenital heart disease (e.g., Fontan procedure) may require 4 J/kg.

(A) **Ventricular fibrillation:** no discernible P, QRS, or T complexes

(B) **PEA:** previously known as **EMD**. Causes—hypoxemia, acidosis, tension pneumothorax, pericardial tamponade, hypovolemia, pulmonary embolism

(C) **Ventricular tachycardia:** more than 3 PVCs in succession

(D) **Aberrant SVT with BBB:** uncommon in children (<10%), assume ventricular tachycardia. If there is no improvement with lidocaine, adenosine can be used to unmask WPW or SVT with block

(E) **Sinus tachycardia:** normal waveform with a rate that exceeds the upper limit of normal for age

(F) **SVT, PAT:** most common pediatric dysrhythmia. Abnormal rate originating proximal to His bundle bifurcation. Rate > 230 bpm. P waves may or may not be discernible, constant R-R interval, normal QRS

(G) **Atrial flutter:** atrial rate 250-500 (usually 300 bpm). P waves are saw tooth, flutter waves; normal QRS, variable ventricular response may be present. Flutter waves are best seen in lead II

(H) **Atrial fibrillation:** P wave present, abnormal QRS, R-R interval irregularly irregular (Ashman's phenomenon)

(I) **Vagal maneuvers:** pharyngeal wall stimulation with nasogastric tube, ice pack to nose and mouth for 15 seconds, Valsalva maneuver if the patient is old enough, or apply carotid massage

(J) **PAC without block:** premature beat, P wave abnormal, normal QRS

PAC with block: similar to above, but may see BBB if conducted; no QRS following P wave if not conducted

(K) **PVC:** premature beat, unrelated P wave, bizarre wide QRS; S-T segment and T wave in a direction opposite to QRS

(L) **Slow rhythms:** treat only if 3rd degree block or symptomatic, i.e., in the presence of CHF or syncope (Stokes-Adams)

(M) **Sinus bradycardia:** normal P wave axis, P-R interval, rate below the lower limit of normal for age. Investigate underlying cause: increased ICP, hypothyroidism, hypothermia, hypoxia, hyperkalemia, gastric distention, drugs

(N) **AVN block:**   1. 1st degree: prolonged P-R interval
2. 2nd degree: Mobitz I (Wenckebach) progressive P-R lengthening prior to a non-conducted P wave
Mobitz II paroxysmal non-conducted P waves
3. 3rd degree: complete AV dissociation, independent atrial and ventricular rates

All above values should be corrected for age unless stated otherwise.

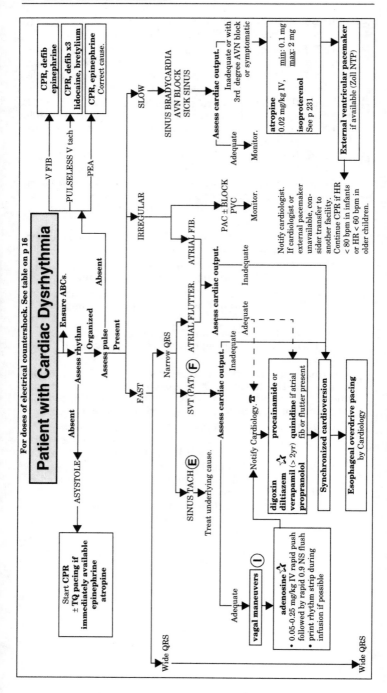

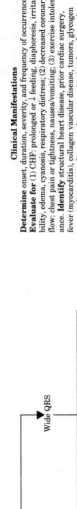

Clinical Manifestations

Determine onset, duration, severity, and frequency of occurrence. **Evaluate for** (1) CHF: prolonged or ↓ feeding, diaphoresis, irritability, edema, cyanosis, respiratory distress; (2) decreased coronary flow: chest pain or tightness, nausea/vomiting; (3) exercise intolerance. **Identify** structural heart disease, prior cardiac surgery, fever (myocarditis), collagen vascular disease, tumors, glycogen storage disease, cardiomyopathy, pre-excitation, hypo/hyperthyroidism. Note medications.

Diagnostics

CBC, differential, platelets, electrolytes, Ca^{+2}, Mg^{+2}, P, 12-lead EKG, chest radiograph. Consider cardiac enzymes, echocardiogram.

✳ Treat unconfirmed SVT as V tach.
Treat confirmed aberrant SVT as SVT.

☆ • Atrial flutter may be unmasked by **adenosine** during its use for the treatment of SVT.
• verapamil and propranolol are (-) inotropic agents and should not be used together.

Wide QRS

Wide QRS

V FIB

Start **CPR.** Defibrillate.

epinephrine

Aberrant SVT ✳

V tach

Assess cardiac output.

Inadequate

Adequate

lidocaine bolus 1 mg/kg IV
lidocaine infusion 20-50 µg/kg/min IV

bretylium 5 mg/kg IV

consider procainamide

Synchronized cardioversion

If no response, Notify Cardiology STAT ☎ _____

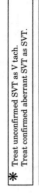

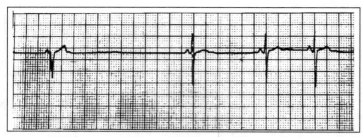

Figure 2-1. *Sinus bradycardia.* Extreme sinus rate variability with P wave rates ranging from 20-75 bpm. The first sinus P wave is followed by a ventricular escape QRS complex.

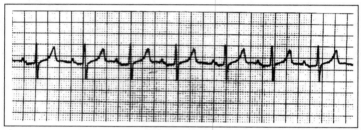

Figure 2-2. *First degree AV block.* Sinus rhythm with all P waves followed by a normal QRS. The P-R interval is prolonged at 0.24 sec, indicating slowed AV conduction. May be seen as a normal response to digoxin or beta-blockade therapy.

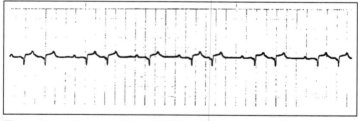

Figure 2-3. *Second degree AV block Wenckebach, Mobitz I.* The preliminary form of 2nd degree AV block with progressive lengthening in the P-R interval before a nonconducted P wave. This example shows 3:2 and 2:1 conduction. This may occur as a normal vagal response in the well-conditioned athlete. May indicate digoxin or beta-blockade toxicity.

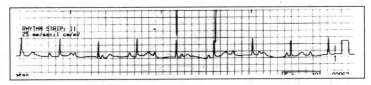

Figure 2-4. *Third degree AV block.* Complete interruption of atrial impulse conduction to the ventricles. The atrial rate is typically faster than the ventricular rate. A normal appearing narrow QRS usually indicates a ventricular escape rhythm high in the conduction system and is usually more stable than a lower origin wide QRS rhythm.

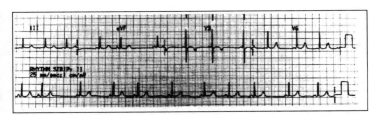

Figure 2-5. *Sinus arrhythmia.* A common finding in infancy and childhood, usually indicating vagal influences on sinus rate. The sinus P wave axis, morphology, and P-R interval are all normal.

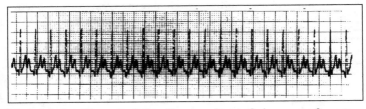

Figure 2-6. *Sinus tachycardia.* Accelerated sinus rate for age. P wave axis, morphology, and P-R interval are normal. Typically "speeds up" and "slows down," rather than accelerating or stopping abruptly.

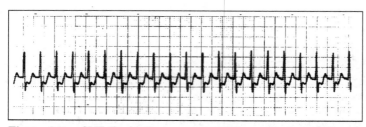

Figure 2-7. *SVT.* Typically a narrow QRS morphology with or without visible P waves at rates > 250 bpm. Also referred to as paroxysmal atrial tachycardia (PAT). Often associated with Wolff-Parkinson-White (WPW) or AV node reentry bypass tracts.

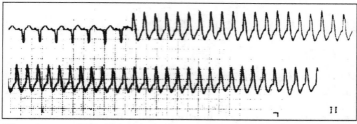

Figure 2.8. *SVT (WPW).* Due to two potential AV connections, the SVT circuit may conduct antegrade to the ventricle via the AV node, giving a narrow QRS (orthodromic conduction). However, a wide QRS resembling ventricular tachycardia may occur if the antegrade conduction utilizes the WPW bypass tract (antidromic conduction). As illustrated, both may occur in the same patient.

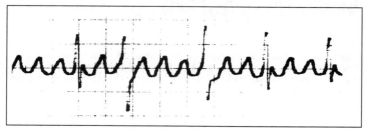

Figure 2-9. *Atrial flutter.* A form of atrial muscle re-entry at a rate approximating 300 bpm. The typical "saw tooth" configuration is often best seen in lead II. This shows variable AV conduction with 4:1, 3:1, and 2:1 conduction.

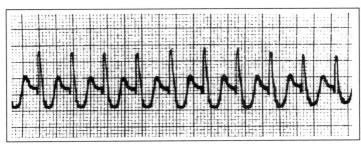

Figure 2-10. *Atrial flutter 2:1.* Due to intrinsic AV node properties, rapid atrial rates of 300 bpm are attenuated, resulting in a common appearance of this tachycardia at 150 bpm. The "saw tooth" pattern is buried in the QRS-T waves.

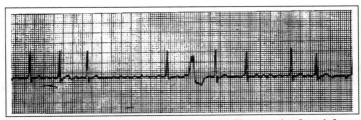

Figure 2-11. *Atrial fibrillation.* A more disorganized atrial muscle tachycardia with nonspecific wavy baseline and variable AV conduction. The commonly associated Ashman phenomenon is illustrated with a wide QRS complex resembling a PVC. This is caused by an atrial impulse conducted to the His-Purkinje system in which the ventricular refractory period has been altered by the preceding long R-R interval.

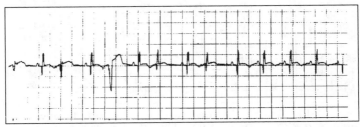

Figure 2-12. *Atrial bigeminy.* A normal sinus P wave followed closely by another, often distorting the preceding T wave, commonly at a fixed "coupled" interval. The resulting QRS may be altered (aberrancy) because of changes in the refractory period and resembles a PVC.

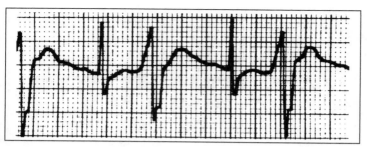

Figure 2-13. *Ventricular bigeminy.* A normal sinus QRS followed by a premature ventricular complex, often at a fixed coupled interval. Depending on the ventricle of origin, a right or left bundle branch block pattern may result.

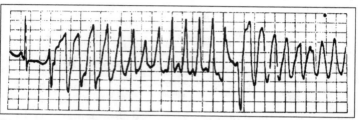

Figure 2-14. *Torsade de Pointes.* A severe form of ventricular tachycardia presenting a variable QRS morphology (multiform) giving the impression of "twisting on the baseline."

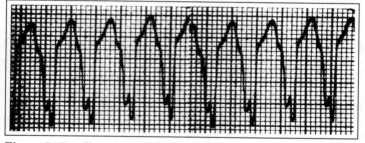

Figure 2-15. *Ventricular tachycardia.* A wide QRS tachycardia often seen with AV dissociation. The rate may vary between 150-300 bpm. Depending on the ventricle of origin, a right or left BBB pattern will occur. Classified as "uniform" or "multiform," depending on the number of distinct QRS patterns.

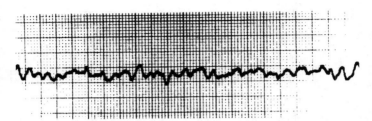

Figure 2-16.   *Ventricular fibrillation*. A nonspecific, irregular baseline electrical activity without organized QRS complexes.

For rhythm strips on hyperkalemia, see p 160.

EKG rhythm strips and commentaries provided courtesy of Peter Karpawich, MD, Division of Cardiology, Children's Hospital of Michigan, Detroit.

"Tet" Spells of Tetralogy of Fallot (TOF)

Katherine Ling-McGeorge

> Paroxysmal hyperpnea of TOF requires immediate recognition and appropriate intervention; severe spells may lead to seizures, CVA, and other CNS complications. There does not appear to be a relationship between the degree of cyanosis at rest and the likelihood of having hypoxic spells.

(A) Peak incidence between 2 and 4 months of age. Usually occurs in the morning. Any event that suddenly lowers the SVR or increases the PVR and produces an increase in right-to-left shunt, e.g., crying, defecation, any increase in activity, feeding, may precipitate the spell.

A decrease in PaO_2 stimulates the respiratory center and results in hyperventilation, thus increasing systemic venous return. In the presence of a fixed RV outflow tract obstruction (pulmonary stenosis), increased systemic venous return results in increased right-to-left shunt (through the VSD), worsening cyanosis. A vicious cycle of hypoxic spells is established.

?Spasm of RVOT
↓SVR, ↑PVR

↑Right-to-Left Shunt

↑Systemic Venous Return

↓PaO_2
↑$PaCO_2$
↓pH

Hyperpnea

Adapted from Park MK. Pediatric Cardiology for Practitioners. p. 117. 1988, With permission from Mosby-Year Book, Inc, St Louis

(B) **Oxygen:** may have limited effect.

(C) **Knee-chest position:** will trap venous blood in the legs, decreasing venous return. May help calm the baby. This position may also increase SVR by blocking arterial blood flow through the femoral arteries.

(D) **Morphine sulfate:** calming effect; breaks cycle of hyperpnea; causes peripheral pooling of unsaturated blood.

(E) **$NaHCO_3$:** reduces the respiratory center-stimulating effect of acidosis.

(F) **Vasoconstrictors:** increase SVR.

(G) **Propranolol:** mechanism of action is not clear, but may act by stabilizing peripheral vascular reactivity, thereby preventing a drop in SVR. Reduces "spasm" of the RV outflow tract.

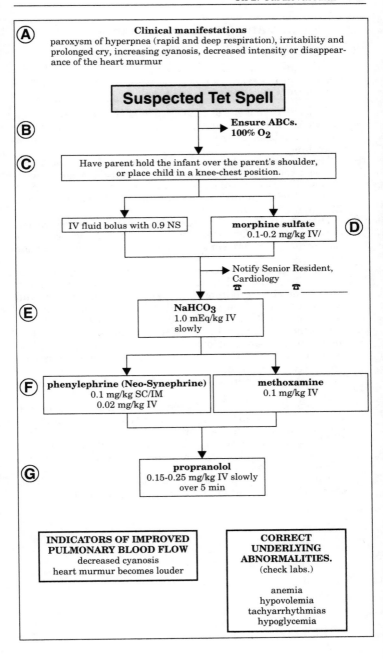

(A)

Clinical manifestations
paroxysm of hyperpnea (rapid and deep respiration), irritability and prolonged cry, increasing cyanosis, decreased intensity or disappearance of the heart murmur

Suspected Tet Spell

(B) → Ensure ABCs.
100% O_2

(C) Have parent hold the infant over the parent's shoulder, or place child in a knee-chest position.

IV fluid bolus with 0.9 NS

morphine sulfate
0.1-0.2 mg/kg IV/ **(D)**

→ Notify Senior Resident, Cardiology
☎_____ ☎_____

(E) $NaHCO_3$
1.0 mEq/kg IV
slowly

(F) **phenylephrine (Neo-Synephrine)**
0.1 mg/kg SC/IM
0.02 mg/kg IV

methoxamine
0.1 mg/kg IV

(G) **propranolol**
0.15-0.25 mg/kg IV slowly
over 5 min

INDICATORS OF IMPROVED PULMONARY BLOOD FLOW
decreased cyanosis
heart murmur becomes louder

CORRECT UNDERLYING ABNORMALITIES.
(check labs.)

anemia
hypovolemia
tachyarrhythmias
hypoglycemia

Hypovolemic and Cardiogenic Shock

Katherine Ling-McGeorge

> A state of circulatory dysfunction with failure to meet the metabolic demands of tissues and end organs. Decreased oxygen delivery. NOT synonymous with hypotension.

(A)   Other labs to consider: comprehensive drug screen, sepsis workup, cortisol level, EKG, echocardiogram, SGOT/ SGPT, amylase, lipase (trauma), alkaline phosphatase or bilirubin

(B)   **Hypovolemic shock:** resulting from decreased effective circulatory volume or preload. History consistent with losses (vomiting, diarrhea, urinary, traumatic). Also observed with conditions leading to third-spacing (burns, GI, nephrotic syndrome)

(C)   **Distributive shock:** resulting from decreased vascular resistance. Observed in spinal shock. Also consider neurogenic, adrenal, septic, anaphylactic, or pharmacologic causes

(D)   **Cardiogenic shock:** resulting from decreased cardiac output. Consider ischemia, myocarditis (child may have a history of viral prodrome), myopathy, dysrhythmias, and congenital cardiac lesions. Unlike hypovolemic shock, the history does not suggest any significant losses

(E)   **Obstructive Shock:** resulting from increased afterload. High index of suspicion is required. Consider cardiac tamponade, pulmonary embolus, tension pneumothorax, and aortic coarctation

(F)   In neonates, dilute $NaHCO_3$ bolus 1:1 with D_5W to decrease hypertonicity.

With acidosis, H^+ is buffered by albumin, elevating free Ca^{+2} levels. As pH normalizes, anticipate **further decrease** in free Ca^{+2} as protein-binding increases. Use $NaHCO_3$ with caution when having difficulty with ventilation, i.e., elevated $PaCO_2$, and in patients with hypernatremia or hypertonicity

(G)   Anemia may be primary or dilutional because of fluid therapy. PRBCs will improve O_2-carrying capacity

Clinical manifestations

GENERAL	diaphoresis, poor skin turgor, cool or warm skin
HEENT	sunken fontanelle or eyes
CVS	tachycardia, weak pulses, delayed capillary refill, cyanosis, pallor/flushed extremities, mottling. **Hypotension is a LATE sign.**
RESP	tachypnea, apnea, Kussmaul respirations, grunting
RENAL	oliguria
CNS	lethargy, agitation

Diagnostics

Ⓐ
Blood	ABG/CBG, CBC, differential, platelets, PT, PTT, type and crossmatch, BUN, creatinine, electrolytes, ionized Ca^{+2}, Mg^{+2}, P, lactic acid
Urine	urinalysis, specific gravity

Patient with Suspected Shock

→ **Ensure ABCs.**

Establish IV or IO access.

Place bladder catheter. ◄ ► Maintain normothermia.

Isotonic crystalloid bolus
20 ml/kg 0.9 NS or LR
IV or IO over 20-30 min
Reassess, may repeat X 1.

Check bedside glucose < 50 mg/dL → **25% dextrose** 1-2 ml/kg IV as $D_{50}W$ diluted 1:1 with 0.9 NS

Supplemental O_2

Reassess patient for disease process.

Ⓑ / Ⓒ / Ⓓ / Ⓔ

HYPOVOLEMIA	**DISTRI-BUTIVE**	**CARDIOGENIC**	**OBSTRUC-TIVE**
Exam: dry	**Exam: Hyper-dynamic**	**Exam: CHF, ↓ perfusion**	*Tension pneumothorax* Thoracentesis (See p 219)
Calculate deficit.	*Sepsis* (See p 94)	*CHF* (See p 10) *Dysrhythmias* (See p 16) *Congenital lesions*	*Cardiac tamponade* Pericardiocentesis (See p 210)
Control losses.	*Adrenal crisis* (See p 38)	• **Prostaglandin E1** 0.05-0.1 µg/kg/min IV (can cause apnea, ↓ BP)	*Pulmonary embolism* Thrombolytics
Replace losses with appropriate fluids:	*Anaphylaxis* (See p 76)	• Start inotropes (see p 231) if indicated.	*LVOTO* Surgical correction
•colloid (plasmanate, albumin)	*Toxins* (See p 96)	•Do not use diuretics at this point.	*Other supportive care*
•O-negative PRBCs		Notify Cardiology. ☎_____	
•crystalloid (0.9 NS, LR)			
DO NOT USE HYPOTONIC FLUIDS for volume expansion.			

Reassess patient, Notify ICU. ☎_____
✳(Continued on p 30)

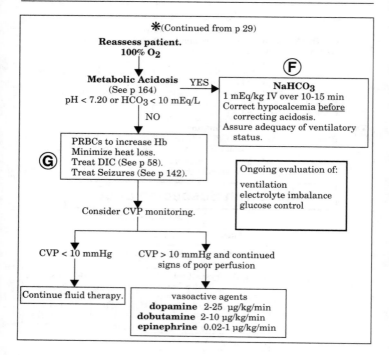

✳(Continued from p 29)

Reassess patient.
100% O$_2$

Metabolic Acidosis   YES → **(F)**
(See p 164)   **NaHCO$_3$**
pH < 7.20 or HCO$_3$ < 10 mEq/L   1 mEq/kg IV over 10-15 min
                            Correct hypocalcemia <u>before</u>
NO   correcting acidosis.
                            Assure adequacy of ventilatory
                              status.

(G) PRBCs to increase Hb
Minimize heat loss.
Treat DIC (See p 58).
Treat Seizures (See p 142).

Ongoing evaluation of:

ventilation
electrolyte imbalance
glucose control

Consider CVP monitoring.

CVP < 10 mmHg   CVP > 10 mmHg and continued
                      signs of poor perfusion

Continue fluid therapy.   vasoactive agents
                            dopamine 2-25 µg/kg/min
                            dobutamine 2-10 µg/kg/min
                            epinephrine 0.02-1 µg/kg/min

Table 2-2.

Agent	Mechanism	Comment
Dopamine	dopaminergic 0.5-6.0 µg/kg/min β agonist 5.0-12.0 µg/kg/min α agonist > 10 µg/kg/min	Limitations: increases myo-cardial O$_2$ consumption.
Dobutamine	β$_1$ inotropic peripheral vasodilation	Decreases SVR.
Epinephrine	β > α β$_1$ inotropic, chronotropic β$_2$ bronchodilation	Limitations: may accelerate ectopic foci, increases myocardial O$_2$ consumption.

Remember Frank-Starling's rule: Ascertain adequate preload before using inotropic agents.
Vasoactive drugs are less effective in acidosis.
For calculation of continuous infusions of vasoactive agents, see p 226.

Notes

Child Abuse

Katherine Ling-McGeorge

According to the National Committee to Prevent Child Abuse*:

Physical abuse: nonaccidental injury to a child that may include severe beatings, burns, strangulation, or human bites

Sexual abuse: sexual exploitation of a child, including rape, incest, fondling of the genitals, exhibitionism, or pornography

Emotional abuse: a pattern of behavior that attacks a child's emotional development and sense of self worth, such as constant belittling, criticizing, insulting, and providing no love, support or guidance

Neglect: failure to provide a child with basic necessities, such as food, clothing, shelter, medical care, education, or proper supervision

Essential to the management of child abuse is the ability to suspect, recognize, evaluate, and treat complications of child abuse.

In 1993, approximately 3 million children nationwide were reported to child protective service agencies. Of these 1,016,000 were confirmed, which included 1,299 fatalities.

Although child neglect and sexual abuse require urgent medical attention, these issues are not addressed in the handbook in the context of emergent care. Children who present with failure to thrive, vaginal bleeding resulting from suspected abusive trauma, and other indications should be hospitalized to undergo further evaluation.

(A) The majority of abused children are < 4 years old. Any condition that interferes with normal parent-child bonding is a risk factor. A child who identifies an adult as the abuser is usually truthful.

Ninety percent of abusive adults are found to be related caretakers. Child abuse crosses all socioeconomic and ethnic groups.

Profile of abused children	Profile of abusive caretakers
prematurity	unrealistic expectations (e.g., toilet training)
multiple birth	young parental age
congenital defect	mental illness
mental retardation	history of abusive childhood
difficult temperament	previous loss of a child
	fear of injury to the child
	domestic violence
	substance use
	crisis situation in abuser's life

(B) Abdominal trauma is the second most common cause of death in battered children. There are usually associated injuries to the skin and head. Note: the abdominal exam may not be reliable in patients with concomitant head injury.

✳(Continued on p 34)

* Child Abuse and Neglect Statistics - April 1994. National Committee to Prevent Child Abuse, 332 S. Michigan Avenue, Suite 1600, Chicago, IL.

Clinical findings

There are characteristic profiles of abused children and their abusive caretakers. Interview the child and all caretakers and witnesses, individually if possible, using nonleading questions.

- suspect: vague explanations · delay in seeking medical care
            alleged self-inflicted injury   no explanation given
            alleged sibling-inflicted injury   varying/changing accounts
            partial confessions   implausible accounts
- note histories that are inconsistent with the injury in severity, distribution, and child's developmental level.

In addition to the organ-specific presentations listed below, the "battered" child may also present with unexplained loss of consciousness, ALTE, shock, or sepsis.

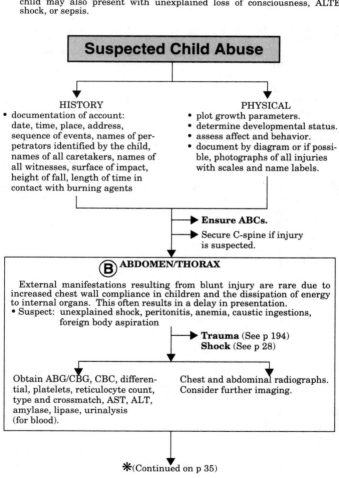

Suspected Child Abuse

HISTORY
- documentation of account:
  date, time, place, address,
  sequence of events, names of per-
  petrators identified by the child,
  names of all caretakers, names of
  all witnesses, surface of impact,
  height of fall, length of time in
  contact with burning agents

PHYSICAL
- plot growth parameters.
- determine developmental status.
- assess affect and behavior.
- document by diagram or if possible, photographs of all injuries
  with scales and name labels.

▶ **Ensure ABCs.**
▶ Secure C-spine if injury
  is suspected.

B ABDOMEN/THORAX

External manifestations resulting from blunt injury are rare due to increased chest wall compliance in children and the dissipation of energy to internal organs. This often results in a delay in presentation.
- Suspect: unexplained shock, peritonitis, anemia, caustic ingestions,
             foreign body aspiration

▶ **Trauma** (See p 194)
  Shock (See p 28)

Obtain ABG/CBG, CBC, differential, platelets, reticulocyte count,
type and crossmatch, AST, ALT,
amylase, lipase, urinalysis
(for blood).

Chest and abdominal radiographs.
Consider further imaging.

✳(Continued on p 35)

✳(Continued from p 32)

> The most common abdominal injuries in order of frequency:
> ruptured liver/spleen
> intestinal perforation
> intramural hematoma of the duodenum, proximal jejunum
> ruptured blood vessels
> pancreatic injury
> kidney/bladder injury
> chylous ascites

From Schmitt BD. The Child with Nonaccidental Trauma. In *The Battered Child*, Helfer RE, Kempe RS. 1987, Chicago: p. 189. The University of Chicago Press. With permission.

(C) Head injury is the most common cause of death in child abuse. In infants with brain trauma, obtain history of feeding, sleeping, and behavior pattern 24-48 hours before presentation.

In a study by Helfer, Slovis, and Black, of 246 falls from the height of a bed or sofa, only 1.2% demonstrated skull fractures. Of the fractures observed, none was bilateral or diastatic.

(D) Ophthalmologic lesions are similar in abuse and in unintentional trauma. Differential diagnoses include: trauma, bleeding disorders, increased intracranial pressure, hypertension. Retinal hemorrhages may be present for > 10 days following an injury.

(E) Differential diagnoses of lesions suggestive of abuse: Mongolian spots, allergic shiners, phytophotodermatitis, erythema marginatum, hypersensitivity, eczema, Henoch Schönlein purpura, Ehlers-Danlos syndrome, and other associated bleeding disorders.

Lesions caused by folk medicine practices: cupping, coin rubbing (cao gio), caida de molera.

	Bruise dating
0- 2 days	tender, swollen
2- 5 days	red, blue, purple
5- 7 days	green
7-10 days	yellow
10-14 days	brown
2- 4 weeks	cleared

From Schmitt BD. The Child with Nonaccidental Trauma. In *The Battered Child*, Helfer RE, Kempe RS. 1987, p 192. Chicago: The University of Chicago Press. With permission.

(F) It is the physicians' responsibility to familiarize themselves with state and local laws governing child abuse, documenting, and reporting.

(G) Differential diagnoses of skeletal abnormalities: osteogenesis imperfecta, congenital syphilis, leukemia, primary bone tumors or metastatic lesions, scurvy, Menke's syndrome (kinky hair syndrome), hyperparathyroidism, birth trauma, and Caffey's disease (infantile cortical hyperostosis)

(H) A "kiddie-gram" is inadequate.

✳(Continued on p 36)

✱(Continued from p 33)

Ⓒ CNS

- common presentations: seizures, altered mental status, coma
- suspect: periorbital ecchymosis, hemotympanum, CSF otorrhea, CSF - rhinorrhea, Battle's sign, bruised or scarred, deformed pinna

Increased ICP (See p 134)
Seizures (See p 142)
Coma (See p 128)

Consider skull radiographs.
- suspect:
  multiple/complex fractures
  fracture width > 5 mm
  massive subgaleal hematoma

Perform funduscopic exam.
Consider:
  retinal detachment Ⓓ
  dislocated lens
  hyphema
  corneal abrasion
  periorbital ecchymosis
  papilledema

- *suspect all retinal hemorrhages.*

Comprehensive drug screen for suspected intentional ingestions

Consider CT scan of the head.
- Suspect:
  chronic subdural hematomas, parafalcine hemorrhage, cerebral edema, hypoxic-ischemic injury

MRI should be considered in detecting and dating subdural hematomas, even if CT was performed initially.

Ⓔ CUTANEOUS LESIONS (document)

- Consider: location, configuration, shape, color, dimensions, differing ages and stages of healing.
- Suspicious sites, i.e., over soft nonbony areas: buttocks, lower back, genitalia, inner thighs, earlobes, cheeks, face, neck

- **Hand marks**
- suspect:
  grab marks or fingertips
  trunk encirclement
  linear marks with finger edge
  slaps
  handprints

- **Contusions suggestive of objects; unnatural in shape (straight or angled edges)**
- suspect:
  looped cord
  belt, buckle
  wire coat hanger
  ankle/wrist ligature

- **Traumatic alopecia**
- Associated with hair pulling
- Suspect subgaleal hematoma

- **Burns**
- suspect:
  more than 2 sites involved
  stocking-glove distribution
  well-demarcated margins
  inconsistent with depth/distribution:
    uniform/symmetric vs.
    arrowhead/splash
  third-degree or full-thickness burns
  reported to result from open flames or
    heating elements
  spared flexion creases resulting from
    withdrawal
  resemble objects: cigarettes, irons, grates
  perineum, buttocks, lower extremities

- **Human bites**
- an intercanine distance > 3 cm indicates
  that the perpetrator is > 8 yr

- **Oral exam**
- suspect:
  frenulum tears/hematomas
  buccal mucosa burns
  lesions in nonambulating

✱(Continued on p 37)

✳(Continued from p 34)

Repeat radiographs should be taken (within 2 weeks) of all sites with previously negative studies, but which are suspected of having sustained traumatic injury.

Ⓘ Siblings of abused children are at a 20% risk of being abused.

Ⓙ Munchausen syndrome by proxy

Common presentations include: seizures, bleeding, altered mental status, apnea, diarrhea, vomiting, fever, and rash.

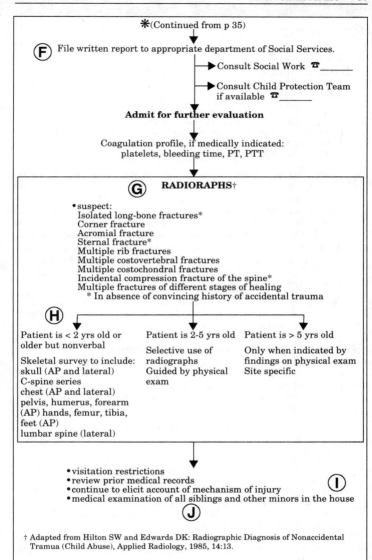

✳(Continued from p 35)

F File written report to appropriate department of Social Services.

➤ Consult Social Work ☎_____

➤ Consult Child Protection Team
if available ☎_____

Admit for further evaluation

Coagulation profile, if medically indicated:
platelets, bleeding time, PT, PTT

G   **RADIORAPHS**†

• suspect:
Isolated long-bone fractures*
Corner fracture
Acromial fracture
Sternal fracture*
Multiple rib fractures
Multiple costovertebral fractures
Multiple costochondral fractures
Incidental compression fracture of the spine*
Multiple fractures of different stages of healing
* In absence of convincing history of accidental trauma

H

Patient is < 2 yrs old or older but nonverbal	Patient is 2-5 yrs old	Patient is > 5 yrs old
Skeletal survey to include: skull (AP and lateral) C-spine series chest (AP and lateral) pelvis, humerus, forearm (AP) hands, femur, tibia, feet (AP) lumbar spine (lateral)	Selective use of radiographs Guided by physical exam	Only when indicated by findings on physical exam Site specific

• visitation restrictions
• review prior medical records
• continue to elicit account of mechanism of injury   **I**
• medical examination of all siblings and other minors in the house

J

† Adapted from Hilton SW and Edwards DK: Radiographic Diagnosis of Nonaccidental
Tramua (Child Abuse), Applied Radiology, 1985, 14:13.

Endocrine

Adrenal Crisis

Kushal Vinod Raghubir

> Adrenal crisis is characterized by a rapid, overwhelming, and potentially fatal adrenocortical insufficiency which may be an intensification of a state of chronic adrenal hypofunction, acute damage to previously normal adrenal glands, or abrupt withdrawal of chronic steroid administration.

(A) In patients with **chronic primary adrenal insufficiency**, suspect acute adrenal crisis with: unexplained fever and hypoglycemia, nausea and vomiting with a history of weight loss and anorexia, abdominal pain, dehydration, shock/hypotension out of proportion to severity of current illness. In **previously normal patients**, consider acute adrenal crisis with the above clinical manifestations, especially in cases of sepsis (meningococcemia, Pseudomonas infection), postoperative (embolic phenomenon), following injury, especially after spinal cord injury.

Note: Hypotension is a late sign of shock. **DO NOT** rely on the presence of low blood pressure as an indicator of shock.

(B)
Classification of adrenal insufficiency

A. Primary adrenal insufficiency
  1. Anatomic destruction of gland (acute and chronic)
     "Idiopathic" atrophy (autoimmune state) usually polyglandular
     Surgical removal, infection (fungal, TB), hemorrhage, infiltration (metastatic)
  2. Metabolic failure in hormone production
     Congenital adrenal hyperplasia, enzyme inhibitors, cytotoxic agents
B. Secondary adrenal insufficiency
  1. Hypopituitarism secondary to pituitary disease
  2. Suppression of hypothalamic-pituitary axis
  3. Exogenous steroids, endogenous steroids from tumor

(C) Glucose may be given as part of the bolus using D_5 0.9 NS, or as a separate bolus of 25% dextrose 1-2 ml/kg, diluted to $D_{12.5}W$ in infants.

(D) Mineralocorticoid deficiency in acute adrenal crisis is treated with correction of electrolytes and **hydrocortisone**. Mineralocorticoids take several days to become fully effective, and parenteral forms are no longer available. **Cortisone acetate** given IM protects the patient in case of loss of IV access. Continuous IV **hydrocortisone** provides the patient with adequate protection in the acute phase.

Use 0.9 NS/D_5 0.9 NS as rehydrating/maintenance solution *until*: (1) laboratory results are obtained, (2) patient is no longer losing electrolytes, and (3) sodium remains stable for 8-12 hours.

*(Continued on p 40)

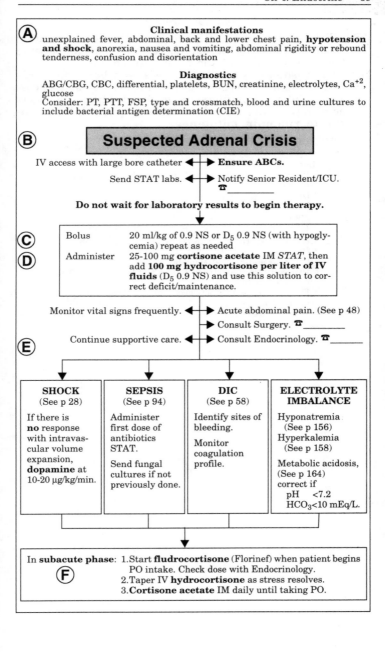

(A) Clinical manifestations
unexplained fever, abdominal, back and lower chest pain, **hypotension and shock**, anorexia, nausea and vomiting, abdominal rigidity or rebound tenderness, confusion and disorientation

Diagnostics
ABG/CBG, CBC, differential, platelets, BUN, creatinine, electrolytes, Ca^{+2}, glucose
Consider: PT, PTT, FSP, type and crossmatch, blood and urine cultures to include bacterial antigen determination (CIE)

(B) ## Suspected Adrenal Crisis

IV access with large bore catheter ◀▶ **Ensure ABCs.**

Send STAT labs. ◀▶ Notify Senior Resident/ICU. ☎ _____

Do not wait for laboratory results to begin therapy.

(C) Bolus — 20 ml/kg of 0.9 NS or D_5 0.9 NS (with hypoglycemia) repeat as needed
(D) Administer — 25-100 mg **cortisone acetate** IM *STAT*, then add **100 mg hydrocortisone per liter of IV fluids** (D_5 0.9 NS) and use this solution to correct deficit/maintenance.

Monitor vital signs frequently. ◀▶ Acute abdominal pain. (See p 48)
▶ Consult Surgery. ☎ _____
Continue supportive care. ◀▶ Consult Endocrinology. ☎ _____
(E)

SHOCK (See p 28)	**SEPSIS** (See p 94)	**DIC** (See p 58)	**ELECTROLYTE IMBALANCE**
If there is **no** response with intravascular volume expansion, **dopamine** at 10-20 µg/kg/min.	Administer first dose of antibiotics STAT. Send fungal cultures if not previously done.	Identify sites of bleeding. Monitor coagulation profile.	Hyponatremia (See p 156) Hyperkalemia (See p 158) Metabolic acidosis, (See p 164) correct if pH <7.2 HCO_3<10 mEq/L.

In **subacute phase**: 1. Start **fludrocortisone** (Florinef) when patient begins
(F) PO intake. Check dose with Endocrinology.
2. Taper IV **hydrocortisone** as stress resolves.
3. **Cortisone acetate** IM daily until taking PO.

✳(Continued from page 38)

(E) Further treatment is based on patient's exacerbating condition. Majority of adrenal crises occur in patients known to have chronic adrenal insufficiency.

(F) Most patients with adrenal crisis need **both** glucocorticoid and mineralocorticoid intake. Ensure that steroid dosage is adjusted in those taking medications that may accelerate hepatic steroid metabolism: **phenytoin, barbiturate, rifampin, mitotane.**

Changes in doses of glucocorticoids related to stress

A. Minor Illness or Stress
   1. Increase glucocorticoid dose 2-3 fold orally for the few days of illness.
   2. DO NOT change mineralocorticoid dose.
   3. No extra supplementation is needed with uncomplicated dental procedures.
   4. If patient is not tolerating PO, notify Endocrinology ☎_____

B. Severe Illness, Stress, or Surgery (when patient is unable to take PO fluids)
   1. Cortisone acetate 25-100 mg IM
   2. Hydrocortisone (Solucortef) 100 mg/L of IV fluid (D_5 0.9 NS) at maintenance rate
   3. Fludrocortisone (Florinef), give with sips of water or by nasogastric tube

---

Notes

Central Diabetes Insipidus

Mary Lieh-Lai

> A syndrome that results from the inability of the neurohypophyseal system to produce a sufficient amount of arginine vasopressin (AVP) to maintain normal renal conservation of free water.

(A)   Causes of DI: idiopathic (50%), either congenital or familial; posthypophysectomy; basal skull fractures or other traumatic brain injury; suprasellar or intrasellar tumors; histiocytosis; vascular lesions and infections

(B)   Differential diagnosis (partial list): psychogenic polydipsia, nephrogenic DI, polyuric phase of acute tubular necrosis, drugs: lithium and demeclocycline

(C)   Continuous intravenous infusion of vasopressin is recommended over **desmopressin (DDAVP)** or IM **pitressin tannate** in oil. The use of continuous IV infusion allows titration of vasopressin according to patient response.

(D)   Hourly laboratory determination may be necessary: urine output (ml/kg/hr) must be monitored, and therapy adjusted accordingly. Hyperglycemia is a frequent side effect of treatment. Serum sodium should not be corrected faster than 0.5-0.75 mEq/L/hr.

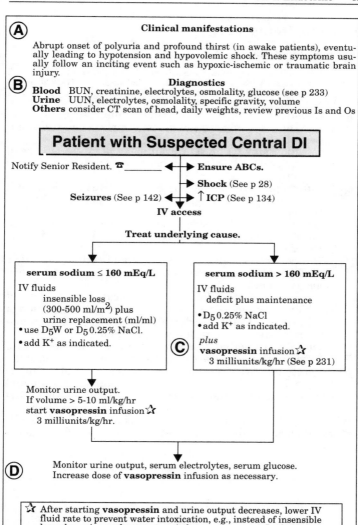

(A)   **Clinical manifestations**

Abrupt onset of polyuria and profound thirst (in awake patients), eventually leading to hypotension and hypovolemic shock. These symptoms usually follow an inciting event such as hypoxic-ischemic or traumatic brain injury.

(B)   **Diagnostics**

Blood BUN, creatinine, electrolytes, osmolality, glucose (see p 233)
Urine UUN, electrolytes, osmolality, specific gravity, volume
Others consider CT scan of head, daily weights, review previous Is and Os

Patient with Suspected Central DI

Notify Senior Resident. ☎_____ ◄─┬─► **Ensure ABCs.**
                                    ├─► **Shock** (See p 28)
Seizures (See p 142) ◄──┬──► **↑ ICP** (See p 134)
                           IV access

Treat underlying cause.

serum sodium ≤ 160 mEq/L
 	
IV fluids
  insensible loss
  (300-500 ml/m^2) plus
  urine replacement (ml/ml)
• use D$_5$W or D$_5$ 0.25% NaCl.
• add K$^+$ as indicated.
	serum sodium > 160 mEq/L
	
	IV fluids
	  deficit plus maintenance
	• D$_5$ 0.25% NaCl
	• add K$^+$ as indicated.
	plus
	(C) **vasopressin** infusion ☆
	  3 milliunits/kg/hr (See p 231)

Monitor urine output.
If volume > 5-10 ml/kg/hr
start **vasopressin** infusion ☆
  3 milliunits/kg/hr.

(D) Monitor urine output, serum electrolytes, serum glucose.
Increase dose of **vasopressin** infusion as necessary.

☆ After starting **vasopressin** and urine output decreases, lower IV fluid rate to prevent water intoxication, e.g., instead of insensible loss plus urine replacement, switch to maintenance fluid rate or less.

Diabetic Ketoacidosis

Maria Asi-Bautista

> Suspect DKA in a child who presents with **hyperglycemia**
> (>300 mg/dl), **ketonemia** (>1:2 dilution), and **acidosis** (pH < 7.20 or
> bicarbonate < 10 mEq/L).

(A) Abdominal pain may sometimes mimic surgical abdomen. The mechanism is unknown. Amylase and transaminases may be elevated.

Infection may be present even if temperature is normal or decreased. Elevated temperature strongly suggests infection.

(B) Fifteen percent may have euglycemic DKA (< 350 mg/dl), e.g., alcoholics and pregnant insulin-dependent diabetic teenagers.

Creatinine is spuriously increased due to interference from acetoacetate. Hyponatremia may be present (see p 156, 233).

(C) If a patient is comatose/stuporous and serum osmolality is < 320 mOsm/L, consider other causes, e.g., toxic ingestions, trauma, etc.

One of the factors frequently implicated as a cause of morbidity and mortality from DKA is the overestimation of fluid deficits. Cerebral edema is induced by the administration of large amounts of hypotonic fluid.

(D) **Insulin is needed to clear ketones.** Continue insulin infusion until ketones are completely cleared from plasma.

(E) Potassium will drop during treatment secondary to (1) urinary losses, (2) increased cell uptake (due to insulin and the correction of metabolic acidosis), (3) dilution from rehydration.

(F) Rapid infusion of sodium bicarbonate has been implicated as one of the factors that can lead to cerebral edema in DKA.

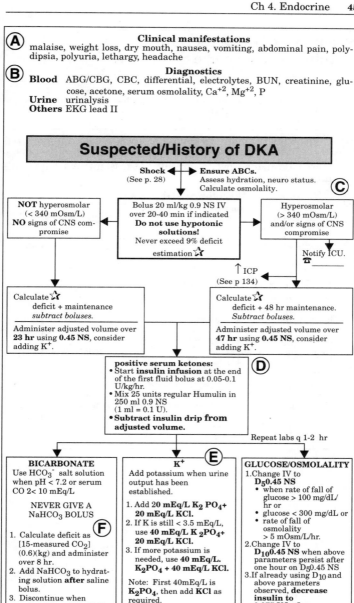

(A) **Clinical manifestations**
malaise, weight loss, dry mouth, nausea, vomiting, abdominal pain, polydipsia, polyuria, lethargy, headache

(B) **Diagnostics**
Blood ABG/CBG, CBC, differential, electrolytes, BUN, creatinine, glucose, acetone, serum osmolality, Ca^{+2}, Mg^{+2}, P
Urine urinalysis
Others EKG lead II

Suspected/History of DKA

Shock ◄──► **Ensure ABCs.**
(See p. 28)   Assess hydration, neuro status.
               Calculate osmolality. **(C)**

NOT hyperosmolar (< 340 mOsm/L) **NO** signs of CNS compromise

Bolus 20 ml/kg 0.9 NS IV over 20-40 min if indicated
Do not use hypotonic solutions!
Never exceed 9% deficit estimation ☆

Hyperosmolar (> 340 mOsm/L) and/or signs of CNS compromise

Notify ICU. ☎ _____

↑ ICP
(See p 134)

Calculate ☆
deficit + maintenance
subtract boluses.

Administer adjusted volume over **23 hr** using **0.45 NS**, consider adding K^+.

Calculate ☆
deficit + 48 hr maintenance.
Subtract boluses.

Administer adjusted volume over **47 hr** using **0.45 NS**, consider adding K^+.

positive serum ketones: **(D)**
• Start **insulin infusion** at the end of the first fluid bolus at 0.05-0.1 U/kg/hr.
• Mix 25 units regular Humulin in 250 ml 0.9 NS (1 ml = 0.1 U).
• **Subtract insulin drip from adjusted volume.**

Repeat labs q 1-2 hr

(E)

BICARBONATE
Use HCO_3^- salt solution when pH < 7.2 or serum CO 2< 10 mEq/L

NEVER GIVE A $NaHCO_3$ BOLUS

1. Calculate deficit as **(F)** [15-measured CO_2] (0.6)(kg) and administer over 8 hr.
2. Add $NaHCO_3$ to hydrating solution **after** saline bolus.
3. Discontinue when serum CO_2 > 15 mEq/L.
4. Do not exceed 77 mEq/L HCO_3, 77 mEq/L Cl⁻, 154 mEq/L Na^+.

K^+
Add potassium when urine output has been established.

1. Add 20 mEq/L $K_2 PO_4$+ 20 mEq/L KCl.
2. If K is still < 3.5 mEq/L, use 40 mEq/L K_2PO_4+ 20 mEq/L KCl.
3. If more potassium is needed, use 40 mEq/L. K_2PO_4 + 40 mEq/L KCl.

Note: First 40mEq/L is K_2PO_4, then add KCl as required.

GLUCOSE/OSMOLALITY
1. Change IV to $D_5 0.45$ NS
   • when rate of fall of glucose > 100 mg/dL/ hr or
   • glucose < 300 mg/dL or
   • rate of fall of osmolality > 5 mOsm/L/hr.
2. Change IV to $D_{10} 0.45$ NS when above parameters persist after one hour on $D_5 0.45$ NS
3. If already using D_{10} and above parameters observed, **decrease insulin to 0.075 U/kg/hr.**

☆ DKA patients may appear more dehydrated than they are, because of hyperventilation (dry lips/mouth) and acidosis (poor myocardial function). Also, older children have less degree of deficit (3, 6, 9%, respectively, for mild, moderate, severe dehydration), as compared to infants.

Syndrome of Inappropriate Antidiuretic Hormone Secretion

Maria Asi-Bautista

> SIADH is characterized by an inappropriate release of ADH in the face of a normovolemic or even hypervolemic state, the clinical features of which include hyponatremia and water intoxication.

(A) Suspected when a patient who is otherwise well hydrated but is at risk for SIADH, suddenly develops oliguria or increased urine specific gravity. Assess intravascular volume status.

(B) Diagnostic criteria for SIADH (See p 233)
- decreased urine volume
- absence of clinical evidence of hypovolemia
- serum osmolality < 270 mOsm/L
- normal BUN
- FE_{Na} > 1
- urine specific gravity > 1.020
- U_{Na} > 30 mEq/L
- urine osmolality > 250 mOsm/L
- BUN:UUN > 1:20

(C) Causes of SIADH (partial list)

Drugs	*vincristine*, vinblastine, carbamazepine, cyclic antidepressants, NSAIDs, morphine
Neoplasm	brain tumors, Hodgkin's disease, acute leukemia, lung cancer
Surgery	anesthesia, surgical stress, spinal fusion
Neurologic	VP shunts, head trauma, hypoxia-ischemia, subarachnoid hemorrhage
Infections	meningitis, pneumonia

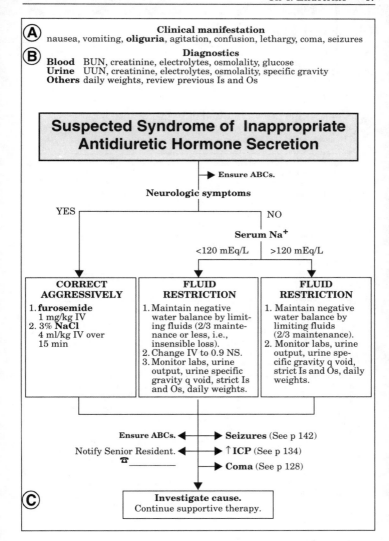

(A) **Clinical manifestation**
nausea, vomiting, **oliguria**, agitation, confusion, lethargy, coma, seizures

(B) **Diagnostics**
Blood BUN, creatinine, electrolytes, osmolality, glucose
Urine UUN, creatinine, electrolytes, osmolality, specific gravity
Others daily weights, review previous Is and Os

Suspected Syndrome of Inappropriate Antidiuretic Hormone Secretion

→ **Ensure ABCs.**

Neurologic symptoms

YES —————————————————————— NO

Serum Na$^+$

<120 mEq/L   >120 mEq/L

CORRECT AGGRESSIVELY	**FLUID RESTRICTION**	**FLUID RESTRICTION**
1. **furosemide** 1 mg/kg IV 2. 3% **NaCl** 4 ml/kg IV over 15 min	1. Maintain negative water balance by limiting fluids (2/3 maintenance or less, i.e., insensible loss). 2. Change IV to 0.9 NS. 3. Monitor labs, urine output, urine specific gravity q void, strict Is and Os, daily weights.	1. Maintain negative water balance by limiting fluids (2/3 maintenance). 2. Monitor labs, urine output, urine specific gravity q void, strict Is and Os, daily weights.

Ensure ABCs. ◄——————► **Seizures** (See p 142)

Notify Senior Resident. ◄——————► ↑**ICP** (See p 134)
☎ _____

——————► **Coma** (See p 128)

Investigate cause.
Continue supportive therapy.

(C)

Gastrointestinal

Acute Abdominal Pain

Jolene Ellis

(A) **Causes of acute abdominal pain by age and location** ☆

Neonate	Infant
Obstruction: atresia, stenosis, duplications Functional obstruction: achalasia, pyloric stenosis, aganglionic megacolon, meconium ileus or plug necrotizing enterocolitis, malrotation, intussusception	gastroesophageal reflux, esophagitis, volvulus, intussusception, Meckel's diverticulum, UTI, hepatitis, ureteropelvic obstruction, tumor

Table 5-1.

	Child	Teenager
Epigastric	peptic ulcer disease, hiatal hernia, esophagitis, pancreatitis	
Periumbilical	appendicitis, cholangitis, inflammatory bowel disease, Meckel's diverticulum, pancreatitis	
LUQ	splenic abscess, splenic sequestration, malignancy	same as child splenic sequestration less common
RUQ	hepatitis, liver abscess, tumor, cholecystitis, cholangitis	
RLQ/LLQ	appendicitis, inflammatory bowel disease	same as child tubo-ovarian abscess, acute ovarian torsion, PID, ectopic pregnancy
Suprapubic	UTI, ureteropelvic obstruction, urolithiasis	Same as child. pregnancy, PID, dysmenorrhea

Causes of peritonitis

(B)

meconium peritonitis acute appendicitis incarcerated hernia inflammatory bowel disease	perforated hollow viscous volvulus intussusception	status post abdominal surgery extension of abscess of solid organ ruptured Meckel's diverticulum

☆Pneumonia may mimic an acute abdomen.
Always obtain and assess chest radiograph.
Abdominal pain may be the first manifestation of an acute abdomen.

Clinical manifestations

acute abdominal pain, localized tenderness, voluntary/involuntary guarding, rebound tenderness, abdominal distention, hypo/hyperactive bowel sounds, history of hematochezia/ melena/hematemesis, Murphy's sign, palpable abdominal or adnexal mass

History: onset, location, referral, quality, associated symptoms/systemic disease; check for history of trauma

Physical exam: vital signs, assess hydration status and overall appearance, lung exam; focused abdominal/pelvic/rectal exam

Diagnostics

Initial lab screen: CBC, differential, platelets, electrolytes, urinalysis, stool guaiac

Additional studies: 3-view abdominal radiograph, chest radiograph, pregnancy test, abdominal ultrasound, liver enzymes/amylase/lipase, type and crossmatch

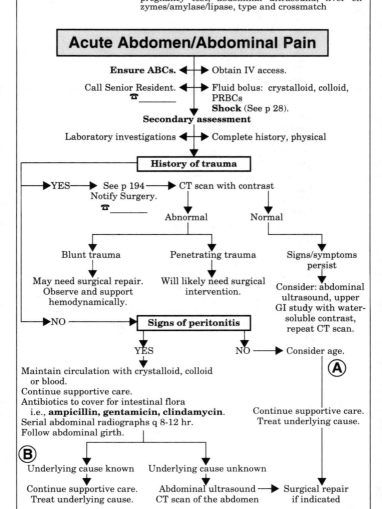

Acute Abdomen/Abdominal Pain

Ensure ABCs. ◄──► Obtain IV access.

Call Senior Resident. ◄──► Fluid bolus: crystalloid, colloid,
☎_____   PRBCs
                           Shock (See p 28).

Secondary assessment

Laboratory investigations ◄──► Complete history, physical

| History of trauma |

──►YES ──► See p 194 ──► CT scan with contrast
        Notify Surgery.
        ☎_____
                        Abnormal   Normal

Blunt trauma   Penetrating trauma   Signs/symptoms
                                            persist

May need surgical repair.   Will likely need surgical   Consider: abdominal
Observe and support   intervention.   ultrasound, upper
hemodynamically.   GI study with water-
                                                         soluble contrast,
──►NO ──► | Signs of peritonitis | repeat CT scan.

                    YES   NO ──► Consider age.

Maintain circulation with crystalloid, colloid   **(A)**
or blood.
Continue supportive care.
Antibiotics to cover for intestinal flora
  i.e., **ampicillin, gentamicin, clindamycin.**   Continue supportive care.
Serial abdominal radiographs q 8-12 hr.   Treat underlying cause.
Follow abdominal girth.

(B)
    Underlying cause known   Underlying cause unknown

    Continue supportive care.   Abdominal ultrasound ──► Surgical repair
    Treat underlying cause.   CT scan of the abdomen   if indicated

Lower Gastrointestinal Bleeding

Joan Less

> True hematochezia: bright red bloody stools
> True melena: tarry black stools
> False hematochezia/melena: seen after ingestion of iron, chocolate,
>   bismuth (PeptoBismol), red Jell-O, red antibiotics, beets, food
>   coloring, licorice
> False positive Hemoccult stool: seen after ingestion of red fruits and
>   meats
> Iron does **not** cause positive Hemoccult stools.

(A) Additional labs to consider: electrolytes, CO_2, BUN, creatinine, ESR, fecal leukocytes

(B) Causes of MILD lower GI bleeding:
hemorrhoids or anal fissure
    (rule out by physical exam)
milk allergy (obtain feeding history)
swallowed maternal blood in a neonate

(C) Causes of MODERATE and SEVERE lower GI bleeding
severe gastroenteritis
infectious colitis
pseudomembranous colitis
Hirschsprung's disease
necrotizing enterocolitis
malrotation with volvulus
Meckel's diverticulum
intussusception
polyps
duplications
inflammatory bowel disease
upper GI sources: peptic ulcer disease,
    gastritis, esophageal varices
others: hemangioma, coagulopathies
Henoch-Schonlein purpura

(D) **Apt-Downey test.** Mix one part of stool or vomitus with 5-10 parts water, and centrifuge. Add 1 ml 0.2 N NaOH to supernatant. Pink color developing in 2-5 minutes indicates fetal hemoglobin. Brown color indicates adult hemoglobin.

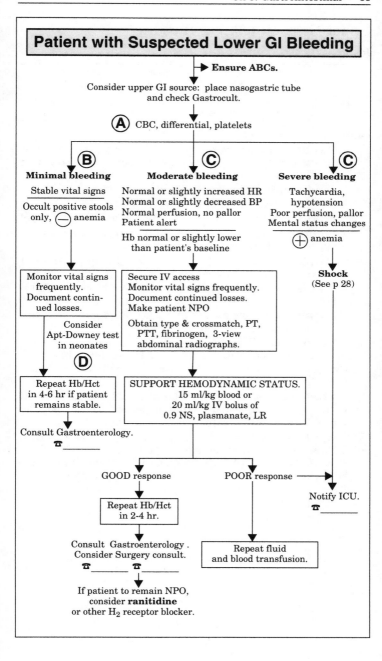

Patient with Suspected Lower GI Bleeding

➤ **Ensure ABCs.**

Consider upper GI source: place nasogastric tube and check Gastrocult.

(A) CBC, differential, platelets

(B)
Minimal bleeding

Stable vital signs

Occult positive stools only, ⊖ anemia

Monitor vital signs frequently.
Document continued losses.

Consider Apt-Downey test in neonates

(D)
Repeat Hb/Hct in 4-6 hr if patient remains stable.

Consult Gastroenterology.
☎_____

(C)
Moderate bleeding

Normal or slightly increased HR
Normal or slightly decreased BP
Normal perfusion, no pallor
Patient alert

Hb normal or slightly lower than patient's baseline

Secure IV access
Monitor vital signs frequently.
Document continued losses.
Make patient NPO

Obtain type & crossmatch, PT, PTT, fibrinogen, 3-view abdominal radiographs.

SUPPORT HEMODYNAMIC STATUS.
15 ml/kg blood or
20 ml/kg IV bolus of
0.9 NS, plasmanate, LR

(C)
Severe bleeding

Tachycardia, hypotension
Poor perfusion, pallor
Mental status changes

⊕ anemia

Shock
(See p 28)

GOOD response

Repeat Hb/Hct in 2-4 hr.

Consult Gastroenterology.
Consider Surgery consult.
☎_____ ☎_____

If patient to remain NPO, consider **ranitidine** or other H$_2$ receptor blocker.

POOR response ➤

Notify ICU.
☎_____

Repeat fluid and blood transfusion.

Upper Gastrointestinal Bleeding

Joan Less

True hematemesis:	coffee-ground material if blood is exposed to gastric acid; bright red blood if bleeding is massive or proximal
False hematemesis:	seen after ingestion of red medications, beets, red juice, red candy

Causes of hematemesis

Swallowed maternal blood. In neonates, Apt-Downey test is used to distinguish maternal blood from neonatal blood.

Mild esophagitis. typically due to gastroesophageal reflux

Mild gastritis. following ingestion of aspirin or ethanol

Mallory-Weiss tear. occurs after forceful vomiting of nonbloody material.

Foreign body ingestion. History is helpful. Protect airway if signs of tracheal compression are observed. If a sharp object is involved, plan endoscopic removal by surgical service.

Esophageal varices. Painless bleeding observed with portal venous hypertension

Peptic ulcer disease. may be either gastric or duodenal. Usually painful. If ulcer penetrates into abdominal cavity, patient may develop shock, peritonitis, and/or pancreatitis.

Stress ulcers. seen in hospitalized, critically ill patients following burns, trauma, sepsis, shock: usually duodenal and multiple; painless.

Ⓐ **Apt-Downey test.** Mix one part of stool or vomitus with 5-10 parts water, and centrifuge. Add 1 ml 0.2 N NaOH to supernatant. Pink color developing in 2-5 minutes indicates fetal hemoglobin. Brown color indicates adult hemoglobin.

Patient with Suspected Upper GI Bleeding

► **Ensure ABCs.**

CBC, differential, platelets

Minimal bleeding

Small volume emesis
Normal HR, BP
No orthostatic
hypotension
Good capillary refill

Normal Hb

Monitor vital signs
frequently.
Document contin-
ued losses.

Make patient NPO.
Place nasogastric
tube.
Check Gastrocult.

Consider
Apt-Downey test
in neonates.

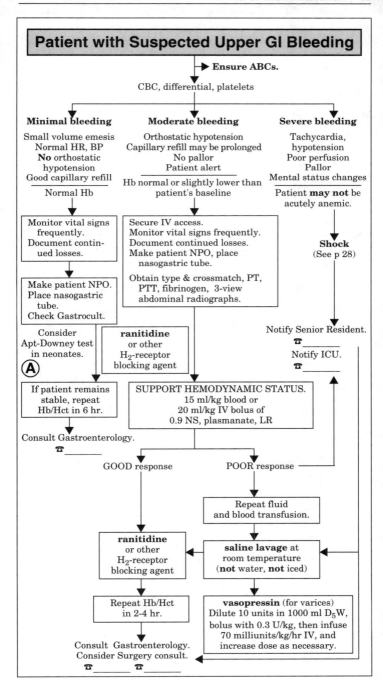

Ⓐ

If patient remains
stable, repeat
Hb/Hct in 6 hr.

Consult Gastroenterology.
☎_____

Moderate bleeding

Orthostatic hypotension
Capillary refill may be prolonged
No pallor
Patient alert

Hb normal or slightly lower than
patient's baseline

Secure IV access.
Monitor vital signs frequently.
Document continued losses.
Make patient NPO, place
nasogastric tube.

Obtain type & crossmatch, PT,
PTT, fibrinogen, 3-view
abdominal radiographs.

ranitidine
or other
H₂-receptor
blocking agent

SUPPORT HEMODYNAMIC STATUS.
15 ml/kg blood or
20 ml/kg IV bolus of
0.9 NS, plasmanate, LR

Severe bleeding

Tachycardia,
hypotension
Poor perfusion
Pallor
Mental status changes

Patient **may not** be
acutely anemic.

Shock
(See p 28)

Notify Senior Resident.
☎_____
Notify ICU.
☎_____

GOOD response   POOR response

Repeat fluid
and blood transfusion.

ranitidine
or other
H₂-receptor
blocking agent

saline lavage at
room temperature
(**not** water, **not** iced)

Repeat Hb/Hct
in 2-4 hr.

vasopressin (for varices)
Dilute 10 units in 1000 ml D₅W,
bolus with 0.3 U/kg, then infuse
70 milliunits/kg/hr IV, and
increase dose as necessary.

Consult Gastroenterology.
Consider Surgery consult.
☎_____   ☎_____

Hematology and Oncology

Anemia

Mary Lieh-Lai

> Anemia is defined as a decreased level of hemoglobin or hematocrit
> more than two standard deviations below the expected mean for an
> individual patient based on age, sex, and physiologic state.
> **Newborn:** 19 ± 2.2 g/dL; falls gradually in the first 8 weeks of life to
> 11.2 ± 4.7 g/dL
> **Older infant/young child:** 11.0-14.0 g/dL
> **Male (puberty):** 14-18 g/dL
> **Female (menarche):** 12-15 g/dL

(A) The signs and symptoms related to severe anemia will depend on the underlying pathology and whether the anemia is chronic or acute. Significant **acute blood loss** can result in a picture of hemodynamic instability and/or shock, while **chronic anemia** may sometimes produce a picture related to a chronic decrease in O_2-carrying capacity with resultant high-output CHF.

(B) Severe anemia accompanied by hemodynamic instability is usually due to acute and significant ($\geq$ 5% total blood volume) blood loss or pooling. Some causes include bleeding from traumatic injury (including child abuse), gastrointestinal hemorrhage, splenic sequestration in patients with sickle cell disease, hemophilia with bleeding episode, DIC with uncontrolled bleeding, intra- or postoperative blood loss.

(C) Causes of anemia resulting from decreased production:
- **Hypochromic, microcytic anemia:** iron deficiency, thalassemia, idiosyncratic, hemosiderosis, congenital atransferrinemia
- **Megaloblastic anemia:** folate deficiency, cobalamine deficiency
- **Normocytic anemia:** chronic renal disease, hypothyroidism, other chronic diseases such as SLE and rheumatoid arthritis.

Marrow infiltration:		leukemias, solid tumors, histiocytosis
Aplasia:	acquired	aplastic, Transient Erythroblastopenia of Childhood
	congenital	Diamond-Blackfan anemia, Fanconi's

✳(Continued on p 56)

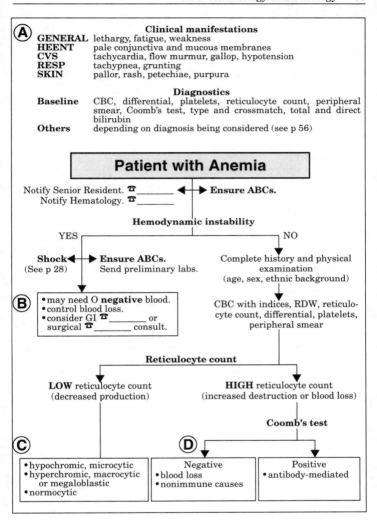

(A) **Clinical manifestations**
GENERAL	lethargy, fatigue, weakness
HEENT	pale conjunctiva and mucous membranes
CVS	tachycardia, flow murmur, gallop, hypotension
RESP	tachypnea, grunting
SKIN	pallor, rash, petechiae, purpura

Diagnostics
Baseline	CBC, differential, platelets, reticulocyte count, peripheral smear, Coomb's test, type and crossmatch, total and direct bilirubin
Others	depending on diagnosis being considered (see p 56)

Patient with Anemia

Notify Senior Resident. ☎_____ ◄──► Ensure ABCs.
Notify Hematology. ☎_____

Hemodynamic instability

YES   NO

Shock ◄──► **Ensure ABCs.**   Complete history and physical
(See p 28)   Send preliminary labs.   examination
                                              (age, sex, ethnic background)

(B)
• may need O **negative** blood.   CBC with indices, RDW, reticulo-
• control blood loss.   cyte count, differential, platelets,
• consider GI ☎_____ or   peripheral smear
  surgical ☎_____ consult.

Reticulocyte count

LOW reticulocyte count   **HIGH** reticulocyte count
(decreased production)   (increased destruction or blood loss)

                                         Coomb's test

(C)   **(D)**
• hypochromic, microcytic | Negative | Positive |
• hyperchromic, macrocytic | • blood loss | • antibody-mediated |
  or megaloblastic | • nonimmune causes | |
• normocytic

✳(Continued from p 54)

Ⓓ Blood loss: acute or chronic
Nonimmune causes:

Intrinsic defects:	Membrane defect	hereditary spherocytosis hereditary elliptocytosis
	Enzyme defect	G6PD, PK, GPI, porphyrias
	Hemoglobinopathies	SS, SC, S-β thalassemia, unstable hemoglobins
Extrinsic defects:	mechanical, chemical, infectious, increased phagocytosis	

Table 6-1.

Condition	Type of Tube	Amount of Blood
Folate deficiency	EDTA (purple top)	3 ml
Cobalamine deficiency	Plain (red top)	3 ml
All membrane defects, e.g., spherocytosis	ACD (yellow top)	5 ml in infants 5-10 ml in older children
Enzyme defects	ACD (yellow top) if not available, use buffered sodium citrate (light blue top)	2 ml (<u>min.</u>)
Hemoglobinopathies	EDTA (purple top)	3 ml

Samples should be collected *prior* to blood transfusion.

Notes

Disseminated Intravascular Coagulation

Michelle Rotta

> Disseminated intravascular coagulation is an acquired or secondary pathologic state characterized by the intravascular consumption of platelets and plasma clotting factors, resulting in thrombi formation and a hemorrhagic state.

(A)   Look for signs of bleeding diathesis or end-organ damage secondary to microvascular thrombosis. Ask about fever, infection, acute gastroenteritis, closed head injury, necrotizing enterocolitis or known coagulopathy.

(B)   Table 6-2.

Test	DIC	Liver Disease	Vitamin K Deficiency	Heparin
PT	↑	↑	↑	↑
PTT	↑	↑	↑	↑
TT	↑	↑	N	↑
Platelets	↓	N or ↓	N	N or ↓
FSP	↑	N or ↑	N	N
D-dimer	positive	negative	negative	negative
β-thromboglobulin Fibrinopeptide A	↑	negative	negative	negative
Fibrinogen	↓	↓	N	N
Antithrombin III	↓	↓	N	N
Factor VIII	↓	N or ↑	N	N
Factor V	↓	↓	N	N
Factor II	↓	↓	↓	N
Protein C and S	↓	↓↓	↓↓	N

N=normal

(C)

	Causes of DIC (partial list)		
shock	liver disease	NEC	asphyxia
sepsis	head injury	transfusion reaction	hemangiomas
	HUS	malignancy (AML)	snake bites

(D)   Others: **topical nitroglycerin** and **heparin** have been reported to be helpful in purpura fulminans.

Ⓐ
	Clinical manifestations
CVS	tachycardia, hypotension, prolonged capillary refill (if associated with shock)
RESP	hemoptysis
GI	jaundice, hematemesis, hematochezia, melena, splenomegaly
RENAL	hematuria, renovascular thrombosis, acute renal failure
CNS	signs of increased ICP, intracranial bleed
HEME	hemolytic anemia
SKIN/MUCOSA	petechiae, purpura, venipuncture or gingival oozing, epistaxis, purpura fulminans, gangrene

Ⓑ
Diagnostics
CBC, differential, platelets, reticulocyte count, peripheral smear, PT, PTT, TT, fibrinogen, FSP, D-dimer assay, type and crossmatch, BUN, creatinine, electrolytes, LFTs, sepsis workup, chest and abdominal radiographs. If indicated: antithrombin III, protein C and S, factors II, V, VIII and assays

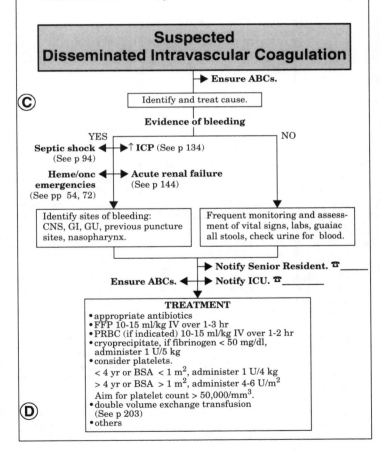

Suspected Disseminated Intravascular Coagulation

➤ **Ensure ABCs.**

Ⓒ
Identify and treat cause.

Evidence of bleeding

YES   NO

Septic shock ◄——► ↑ **ICP** (See p 134)
(See p 94)

Heme/onc ◄——► **Acute renal failure**
emergencies   (See p 144)
(See pp 54, 72)

Identify sites of bleeding: CNS, GI, GU, previous puncture sites, nasopharynx.	Frequent monitoring and assessment of vital signs, labs, guaiac all stools, check urine for blood.

➤ **Notify Senior Resident.** ☎ _____

Ensure ABCs. ◄——► **Notify ICU.** ☎ _____

TREATMENT
- appropriate antibiotics
- FFP 10-15 ml/kg IV over 1-3 hr
- PRBC (if indicated) 10-15 ml/kg IV over 1-2 hr
- cryoprecipitate, if fibrinogen < 50 mg/dl, administer 1 U/5 kg
- consider platelets.
  < 4 yr or BSA < 1 m^2, administer 1 U/4 kg
  > 4 yr or BSA > 1 m^2, administer 4-6 U/m^2
  Aim for platelet count > 50,000/mm^3.
- double volume exchange transfusion (See p 203)
- others

Ⓓ

Hemophilia Emergencies

Sunita Sarin

> Hemophilia is a hereditary bleeding disorder characterized by a factor deficiency (factor VIII or factor IX) which results in uncontrolled bleeding.

(A)

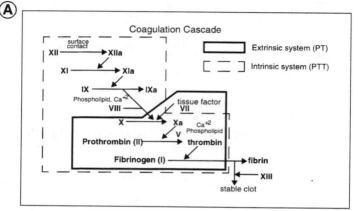

Figure 6-1.

(B) Mucous membrane bleeding is most common in toddlers; often a single dose of factor will result in cessation of bleeding. However, the clot can easily be dislodged, and further bleeding may occur. Consider antifibrinolytic agents such as **epsilon aminocaproic acid** (Amicar), **tranexamic acid**.

(C) Acute hemarthroses should be suspected if a child with hemophilia starts to limp, has joint swelling or pain, or is complaining of peculiar tingling sensation in the joint. Hemarthroses should be treated immediately in an attempt to stop bleeding and prevent accumulation of large amounts of blood in the joint space, which can be irritating. Synovial proliferation into the joint space can lead to repeated trauma of the highly vascular synovial membrane projections, which leads to rebleeding.

(D) Intramuscular bleeding usually presents with a history of traumatic injury. Common sites include the thighs, calf, forearm, and iliopsoas muscle. The affected muscle mass will appear hard, swollen, and tender.

BEWARE of Compartment syndrome that can occur with extensive soft tissue bleeding in the extremities. This can compromise circulation in the involved space. A surgical consultation is needed emergently for possible fasciotomy. Immediate treatment with factor, application of cold compress, and elevation of the affected extremity is necessary while awaiting surgical evaluation.

Clinical manifestations
shock, hypotension, respiratory distress, mental status changes, mucous membrane bleeds, joint or muscle swelling and/or pain

Diagnostics
CBC, differential, platelets, peripheral smear, PT, PTT, TT, fibrinogen, type and crossmatch inhibitor assay (in life-threatening bleeds, prior to administration of factors)

Hemophilia with Bleeding

Ensure ABCs. ◄───► **Shock** (See p 28)

Notify Senior Resident, ICU. ◄───► ↑ **ICP** (See p 134)

Notify Hematology. ☎_____ ◄───

Determine site of bleeding

If **intracranial bleeding** is suspected, _prior to imaging_, immediately administer:

factor VIII	(Recombinate, Kogenate)	50 U/kg IV (hemophilia A)
factor IX	(Mononine, Alphanine SD)	50 U/kg IV (hemophilia B)

☆ • Page Neurosurgery STAT. ☎_____
• Page Radiology STAT. ☎_____
• Page Hematology STAT. ☎_____

Ensure ABCs. ◄─ ✴(Continued on p 62)

(Continued on p 62)

(B)

MUCOUS MEMBRANE
☆

• **factor VIII**
(Recombinate, Kogenate)
20 U/kg IV initially, then
20 U/kg q 12 hr x 3-5 days
• **factor IX** (Mononine)
30 U/kg IV initially then
30 U/kg q 12 hr x 3-5 days

Adjuvant therapy

• **aminocaproic acid**
(Amicar) 50 mg/kg/dose
PO q 6 hr

or

• **tranexamic acid**
25 mg/kg/dose PO q 8 hr

(C)

ACUTE HEMARTHROSES
☆

• **factor VIII**
(Recombinate, Kogenate)
20 U/kg IV initially, usually does not require
repeat dose.

• **factor IX** (Mononine)
30 U/kg IV

NOTE: Treat immediately.
By the time the child
seeks medical attention, a
significant amount of
time has elapsed.

(D)

INTRAMUSCULAR
☆

• **factor VIII**
(Recombinate, Kogenate)
30 U/kg IV then 20 U/kg
q 12 hr until affected
muscle mass is soft and
decreased in size

• **factor IX** (Mononine)
30-40 U/kg IV then
30 U/kg q 12 hr

• **with** Compartment syndrome page Surgery STAT.
☎_____

☆ **NOTE:** In the presence of factor VIII Inhibitor, give
first dose **FEIBA or Autoplex** 75 units/kg/dose IV
STAT and consult Hematology for further dosing.
☎_____

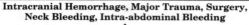

✱(Continued from p 61)

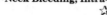

Intracranial Hemorrhage, Major Trauma, Surgery, Neck Bleeding, Intra-abdominal Bleeding ☆

- **Factor VIII** (Recombinate, Kogenate) 50 U/kg IV then 25-30 U/kg q 8-12 hr or as continuous infusion 3-4 U/kg/hr
- **factor IX** (Mononine) 50 U/kg IV then 20-25 U/kg q 12 hr or as continuous infusion 4 U/kg/hr
- Monitor response daily.

Following surgery, patients with hemophilia must be monitored closely for oozing. They may need additional factor infusion. If bleeding or oozing persists, page Hematology STAT. ☎ _____

Available products

Hemophilia A (VIII deficiency)
- *do not use cryoprecipitate* (increased risk of hepatitis)
- **factor VIII concentrate** immunoaffinity purified factor VIII (do not use in previously untreated patients) Monoclate P, Hemofil M
- **recombinant factor VIII** (Recombinate, Kogenate) - preferred product
- **desmopressin (DDAVP)** 0.3 µg/kg IV diluted in 50 ml 0.9 NS administer over 10-15 min
  Use only for mild hemophilia A with no life-threatening bleed.

Hemophilia B (IX deficiency)
- **do not use factor IX complex concentrate (PCC)** in previously untreated patients
- **do not use fresh frozen plasma** — not heat treated, so may not be virus-free.
- Mononine, Alphanine SD — preferred products

Inhibitor antibodies may develop to the deficient factor. Present in 20-25% of patients with severe hemophilia A and in 3% of patients with severe hemophilia B
- **activated PCC** (FEIBA or Autoplex) 75 units/kg/dose IV
- **porcine factor VIII** (Hyate C)
- **recombinant VIIa** — available only on the basis of *compassionate* use

Notes

Neutropenia with Fever

Maria Asi-Bautista

(A) Neutropenic patients are more likely to have cellulitis than abscesses. Also, because of their impaired inflammatory response, typical signs of inflammation/infection may not be seen. As such, **erythema** may be the most important clue to the presence of infection.

Pay particular attention to the (1) history of transfusions, (2) nature of drug therapy: list of drugs, duration of treatment, timing and dose, (3) use of analgesics, antipyretics and antibiotics, and (4) recent surgery.

Visual inspection of perianal area is necessary, but digital manipulation should not be performed. The presence of a perirectal abscess in a neutropenic patient is presumed to be due to *Pseudomonas* until proven otherwise.

(B) *Ideally*, cultures should be drawn prior to the first dose of antibiotic, but never withhold antibiotics because of the inability to obtain cultures.

Ensure that specimens are labeled properly, particularly when blood cultures are drawn from several sites. Generally, if the cause of infection is bacterial, organisms will grow in 90% of blood cultures within 72 hours of incubation.

Positive cultures from catheters can sometimes reflect infection in or around the catheter, and results should be compared with peripheral blood cultures before making the diagnosis of bacteremia. Additionally, cultures from mucosal surfaces, respiratory secretions and skin surfaces should be interpreted with caution as they may represent bacterial colonization or overgrowth.

(C) Infectious diseases are the most common cause of neutropenia in children.

Table 6-3.

Drugs that can cause neutropenia (partial list)	
Antibiotics	aminoglycosides, amphotericin, cephalosporins, penicillin, sulfa, trimethoprim-sulfamethoxazole
Anticonvulsants	barbiturates, carbamazepine, clonazepam, ethosuximide, phenytoin
Anti-inflammatory agents	aspirin, ibuprofen, indomethacin, naproxen, penicillamine
Others	acetazolamide, *antineoplastics*, imipramine, procainamide, propranolol, thiazides

*(Continued on p 66)

(A)

Clinical manifestations

HEENT	mucositis, stomatitis, gingivitis, pharyngitis, recurrent otitis media, pain over sinuses
CVS	hypotension, increasing fluid requirements
RESP	recurrent pneumonias
GI	diarrhea, abdominal pain, dysphagia, hepatosplenomegaly
GU	oliguria, dysuria
CNS	signs of increasing ICP, seizures, headache, mental status changes
HEME	associated DIC, thrombocytopenia, anemia, hemolysis
SKIN	macules, pustules, maculopapules, vesicles, abscesses (especially perirectal, groin), ulcers, infarcts
EXT	localized pain or tenderness, erythema

(B)

Diagnostics

Blood	ABG/CBG, CBC, differential, platelets, reticulocyte count, peripheral smear, BUN, creatinine, electrolytes, glucose, blood cultures (include specimens from each catheter port/lumen). Consider: coagulation profile, LFTs
Urine	urinalysis, culture, CIE.
Others	chest radiographs, culture of respiratory secretions, stool cultures, CSF culture and CIE, wound aspirate culture. Consider bone marrow aspiration, abdominal ultrasound, bone scan

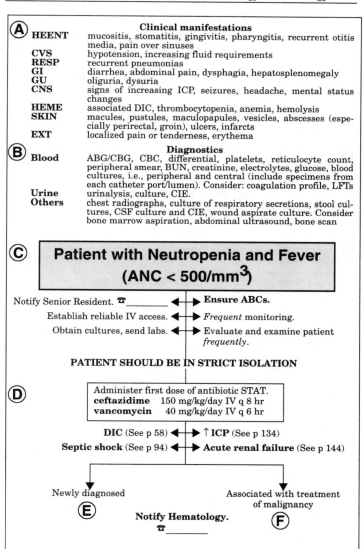

(C)

Patient with Neutropenia and Fever (ANC < 500/mm³)

Notify Senior Resident. ☎_____ ◄─► **Ensure ABCs.**

Establish reliable IV access. ◄─► *Frequent* monitoring.

Obtain cultures, send labs. ◄─► Evaluate and examine patient *frequently*.

PATIENT SHOULD BE IN STRICT ISOLATION

(D)

Administer first dose of antibiotic STAT.
ceftazidime 150 mg/kg/day IV q 8 hr
vancomycin 40 mg/kg/day IV q 6 hr

DIC (See p 58) ◄─► ↑ **ICP** (See p 134)

Septic shock (See p 94) ◄─► **Acute renal failure** (See p 144)

Newly diagnosed
(E)

Associated with treatment of malignancy
(F)

Notify Hematology.
☎_____

*(Continued from p 64)

(D) Common pathogens encountered: *Staphylococcus, Escherichia coli, Klebsiella pneumoniae, Pseudomonas.*

Specific agents may be added in cases of:

diffuse lung infiltrate	**trimethoprim-sulfamethoxazole**
areas of lung consolidation	**erythromycin**
catheter sepsis	**vancomycin**
diarrhea, abdominal pain	**metronidazole**

(E) Patients should be carefully evaluated for evidence of other hematologic involvement.

(F) **Table 6-4. INFECTIONS MIMICKING NEOPLASMS: DIAGNOSTIC CONSIDERATIONS***

Findings	Causative organisms
Brain metastases	*Nocardia asteroides, Toxoplasma gondii*
Budd-Chiari syndrome	*Mucor* spp., *Aspergillus*
Intestinal obstruction	*Strongyloides intestinalis, Entameoba histolytica*
Nephrotic syndrome	*Mucor* spp., *Aspergillus*
Renal vein thrombosis	Gram-negative bacilli
Obstructive nephropathy	*Candida*
Oculomotor palsy	*Zygomycosis*
Pulmonary nodules	*Histoplasma capsulatum, Pneumocystis*
Superior vena cava syndrome	Histoplasma capsulatum

Causes of Recurrent or Persistent Fever in Patients with Negative Bacterial and Fungal Cultures*

adrenal insufficiency	graft-versus-host disease
anicteric viral hepatitis	hematomas, infected or uninfected
catheter-associated infection (including candidiasis)	drug fever
CHF	other viral infections
cryptic abscess	pulmonary emboli
cytomegalovirus infection (with or without hepatitis)	splenic infarct
Epstein-Barr virus infection	tuberculous or other granulomatous disease
	underlying disease

*From Young LS. Fever and Septicemia. In Rubin RH, Young LS (eds), *Clinical Approach in the Compromised Host.* New York: Plenum Publishing Corporation, 1988, pp 75–111. With permission.

Notes

Sickle Cell Disease

Michelle Rotta

> **Sickle cell disease:**   hemoglobinopathies characterized by the formation of sickled red cells in response to deoxygenation.
> **Sickle cell anemia:**   substitution of valine for glutamine in the 6th amino acid position of the β chain. Others: HbSC, sickle-thalassemia combinations. All sickle cell patients should be considered as immuno-compromised hosts.

(A)   **Table 6-5.**

Syndrome	Hematocrit %	Reticulocyte %	MCV (mean)	Electro-phoresis	Spleno-megaly
SS	18-28	12-25	86	S↑ F↑ A$_2$↑	child - yes adult - no
SC	30-36	5-10	77	S↑ C↑	yes
Sβ^0 thal	20-30	10-15	66	S↑ F↑ A$_2$↑	yes
Sβ$^+$ thal	30-36	3- 6	70	S↑ F↑ A$_2$↑ A↓	yes
SSα thal (α$^-$ α$^-$)	25-30	5-10	70	S↑ F↑ A$_2$↑	variable

Normal Hb = 90-95%, A$_2$ 3%, F up to 2%

Therapy

1. **Stabilization:** ABCs, treat shock, frequent reassessment
2. **Hydration:** 1.5-2.0X maintenance, monitor volume status. Pump failure and renal concentrating defects are often encountered.
3. **Liberal pain control:** relaxes patient, enhances pulmonary toilet. Use with caution when abdominal symptoms present. Do not make the patient ask for medications. Consider patient-controlled analgesia (PCA pump). PCA is contraindicated in patients with respiratory distress.
   acetaminophen with codeine
   morphine 0.1 mg/kg/dose IM/SC q 3-4 hr then 0.6 mg/kg/dose PO

(B)   4. **Antibiotics:** must provide coverage for encapsulated organisms (*S. pneumoniae, H. influenzae*). Other organisms: *Chlamydia, Mycoplasma, Staphylococcus, Salmonella* (osteomyelitis). Suggested coverage:
   - < 8-10 yr   cefuroxime ± erythromycin
   - > 8-10 yr   penicillin ± erythromycin
      consider cefotaxime for gram-negative coverage or resistant *S. pneumoniae*.
5. **Partial exchange transfusion:** Indications: CVA, splenic sequestration, acute chest syndrome, pneumonia, hypoxia, prolonged priapism (> 4-6 hr), severe/prolonged pain crisis, pre-op, contrast study. See p 209.
6. **Straight transfusion:** 12 ml/kg PRBC. Indications: aplastic crisis, shock, splenic sequestration.

✳(Continued on p 70)

Clinical manifestations

History   Ask about fever, respiratory, or neurologic symptoms, pain (typical or atypical). In patients with known sickle cell disease, check Hb type, usual Hb and reticulocyte count; history of previous transfusions or ICU admissions (and indications), immunization status.

Physical exam   Signs of infection, fever, tachycardia, hypotension, hepatosplenomegaly, abdominal pain, bone pain, neurologic deficits, mental status changes, jaundice.

Diagnostics

(A) CBC, differential, platelets, reticulocyte count, peripheral smear, type and crossmatch/hold, Hb solubility, Hb electrophoresis (if indicated)

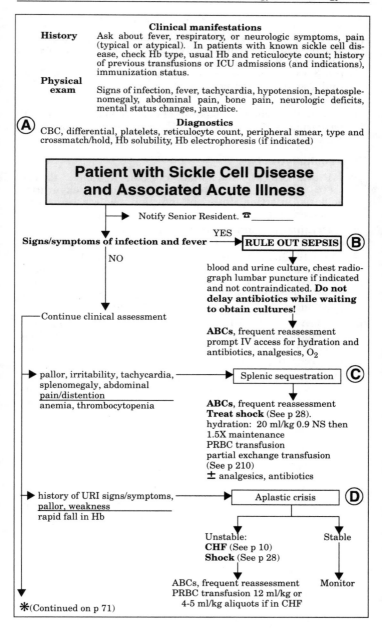

Patient with Sickle Cell Disease and Associated Acute Illness

→ Notify Senior Resident. ☎ _____

Signs/symptoms of infection and fever —— YES ——→ **RULE OUT SEPSIS** **(B)**

NO

blood and urine culture, chest radiograph lumbar puncture if indicated and not contraindicated. **Do not delay antibiotics while waiting to obtain cultures!**

ABCs, frequent reassessment prompt IV access for hydration and antibiotics, analgesics, O_2

—Continue clinical assessment

→ pallor, irritability, tachycardia, —→ Splenic sequestration **(C)**
splenomegaly, abdominal pain/distention
anemia, thrombocytopenia

ABCs, frequent reassessment
Treat shock (See p 28).
hydration: 20 ml/kg 0.9 NS then 1.5X maintenance
PRBC transfusion
partial exchange transfusion
(See p 210)
± analgesics, antibiotics

→ history of URI signs/symptoms, —→ Aplastic crisis **(D)**
pallor, weakness
rapid fall in Hb

Unstable: Stable
CHF (See p 10)
Shock (See p 28)

ABCs, frequent reassessment   Monitor
PRBC transfusion 12 ml/kg or
4-5 ml/kg aliquots if in CHF

✳(Continued on p 71)

✳(Continued from 68)

(C)   **Splenic sequestration:**   massive RBC sequestration in spleen; acute drop in Hb > 2 g/dl, reticulocytosis; signs and symptoms of intravascular volume depletion. 20-25% recurrence rate, most common age 10-27 months. HbSC, Sβ thalassemia—continued risk secondary to incomplete autosplenectomy.

(D)   **Aplastic crises:**   cessation of erythropoiesis; seen with parvovirus B19, also EBV, CMV; spontaneous resolution in 1-2 weeks, may require supportive transfusions.

Vaso-occlusive crises

(E)   **Pain:**   typically abdominal, long bone and back; dactylitis (6-12 months old). Precipitants: hypoxia, dehydration, acidosis, infection. Rule out infection, cholecystitis, acute abdomen, and osteomyelitis

(F)   **Priapism:**   painful erection, needs immediate transfusion. Primarily seen in adolescents. Commonly recurs.

(G)   **Acute chest syndrome** (pneumonia/infarct):   may be associated with *S. pneumoniae.*   Consider *Mycoplasma, Chlamydia,* or TB if there is no improvement with appropriate treatment for common bacterial infections. Patients need adequate analgesia to help facilitate pulmonary toilet

(H)   **CVA:**   seen in 5-15% of HbSS patients. If strongly suspected, patient needs an emergent non-contrast head CT. Usually due to thrombosis in children, hemorrhage in adults; high recurrence rate

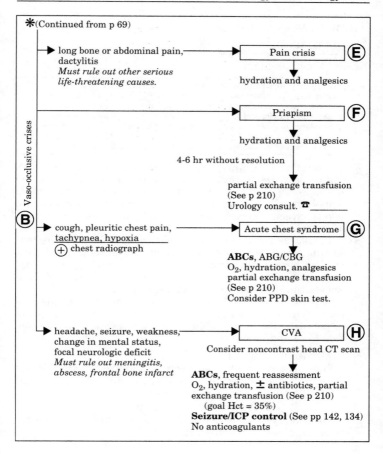

✱(Continued from p 69)

Vaso-occlusive crises **B**

→ long bone or abdominal pain, dactylitis
Must rule out other serious life-threatening causes. ————→ Pain crisis **E**

hydration and analgesics

————————————————————→ Priapism **F**

hydration and analgesics

4-6 hr without resolution

partial exchange transfusion (See p 210)
Urology consult. ☎_____

→ cough, pleuritic chest pain, tachypnea, hypoxia
⊕ chest radiograph ————→ Acute chest syndrome **G**

ABCs, ABG/CBG
O_2, hydration, analgesics
partial exchange transfusion (See p 210)
Consider PPD skin test.

→ headache, seizure, weakness, change in mental status, focal neurologic deficit
Must rule out meningitis, abscess, frontal bone infarct ————→ CVA **H**

Consider noncontrast head CT scan

ABCs, frequent reassessment
O_2, hydration, ± antibiotics, partial exchange transfusion (See p 210)
(goal Hct = 35%)
Seizure/ICP control (See pp 142, 134)
No anticoagulants

Tumor Lysis Syndrome
Hyperuricemia

Kushal Vinod Raghubir

> A group of biochemical abnormalities (hyperuricemia, hyperkalemia, and hyperphosphatemia with hypocalcemia) that arises from the rapid release of intracellular metabolites in quantities that exceed the excretory capacity of the kidneys; associated with massive destruction of a large number of rapidly proliferating neoplastic cells; predominantly seen in tumors with a large cell burden that are very sensitive to chemotherapeutic agents, e.g., T-cell leukemia, B-cell lymphoma.

(A) Excretion is compromised if renal function is poor, leading to progressive precipitation of uric acid crystals in the distal renal tubules, obstructive uropathy, and azotemia. This form of renal failure usually occurs when serum urate levels exceed 20 mg/dl, but may occur with levels as low as 10 mg/dl.

(B) Measures should be instituted in every case of acute leukemia/lymphoma prior to commencing specific treatment (chemotherapy/radiation) regardless of level of uric acid, but especially in patients with large tumor load (high leukocyte count or massive organomegaly).

(C) **Allopurinol** is a competitive inhibitor of xanthine oxidase. This enzyme catalyzes the final steps of degradation of purines to uric acid. May cause a hypersensitivity reaction heralded by a rash.

(D) Maintain urine pH 7.0–7.5.
Note: 1. Severe alkalosis decreases ionized calcium levels secondary to increased protein binding, and therefore should be avoided.
2. See hyperphosphatemia (p 74).

(E) Hemodialysis is 10-20 times more effective than peritoneal dialysis in removing uric acid.

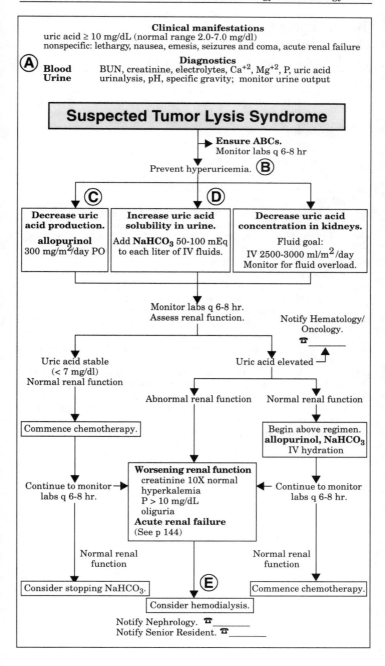

Clinical manifestations
uric acid ≥ 10 mg/dL (normal range 2.0-7.0 mg/dl)
nonspecific: lethargy, nausea, emesis, seizures and coma, acute renal failure

(A)

Diagnostics

Blood	BUN, creatinine, electrolytes, Ca^{+2}, Mg^{+2}, P, uric acid
Urine	urinalysis, pH, specific gravity; monitor urine output

Suspected Tumor Lysis Syndrome

Ensure ABCs.
Monitor labs q 6-8 hr

Prevent hyperuricemia. **(B)**

(C)

Decrease uric acid production.

allopurinol
300 mg/m^2/day PO

(D)

Increase uric acid solubility in urine.

Add **NaHCO$_3$** 50-100 mEq to each liter of IV fluids.

Decrease uric acid concentration in kidneys.

Fluid goal:
IV 2500-3000 ml/m^2/day
Monitor for fluid overload.

Monitor labs q 6-8 hr.
Assess renal function.

Notify Hematology/
Oncology.
☎ _____

Uric acid stable
(< 7 mg/dl)
Normal renal function

Uric acid elevated

Commence chemotherapy.

Abnormal renal function

Normal renal function

Continue to monitor
labs q 6-8 hr.

Begin above regimen.
allopurinol, NaHCO$_3$
IV hydration

Worsening renal function
creatinine 10X normal
hyperkalemia
P > 10 mg/dL
oliguria
Acute renal failure
(See p 144)

Continue to monitor
labs q 6-8 hr.

Normal renal
function

Consider stopping NaHCO$_3$.

(E)

Normal renal
function

Commence chemotherapy.

Consider hemodialysis.

Notify Nephrology. ☎ _____
Notify Senior Resident. ☎ _____

Tumor Lysis Syndrome Hyperphosphatemia (and Associated Hypocalcemia)

Kushal Vinod Raghubir

> When the $[Ca^{+2}]$ X [P] ion product exceeds 60, precipitation of $CaPO_4$ crystals in the microvasculature and renal tubules occurs, causing renal and tissue damage. Patients predisposed to tumor lysis syndrome include the following:
> - patients with large tumor burdens, especially lymphoproliferative lesions
> - patients with poor renal function (phosphorus is cleared by glomerular filtration)

(A)   Chvostek's sign may be elicited prior to the occurrence of other listed symptoms.

(B)   Routine labs in all cases of newly diagnosed malignancies. In lymphoproliferative malignancies, monitor q 6-8 hr.

(C)   Phosphorus is normally reabsorbed, but when the reabsorption maximum is exceeded, excretion depends on glomerular filtration. Diuretics may assist by influencing the reabsorption maximum.

(D) $NaHCO_3$ infusion: $CaPO_4$ crystals are less soluble with a urine pH > 6, therefore in the face of severe hyperphosphatemia, alkalinization should be discontinued.

(E)   Effects of orally administered $Al(OH)_3$ are unpredictable.

(F)   Must take into account that increases in Ca^{+2} in patients with hyperphosphatemia may cause further precipitation of $CaPO_4$.

(G)   Treat Ca^{+2}-induced bradycardia by decreasing Ca^{+2} infusion and if necessary, by administering **atropine** 0.01 mg/kg IV.

(H)   If hypomagnesemia is present, ionized calcium level will remain abnormal despite Ca^{+2} administration, until hypomagnesemia is corrected.

(I)   Hemodialysis is the preferred mode of therapy.

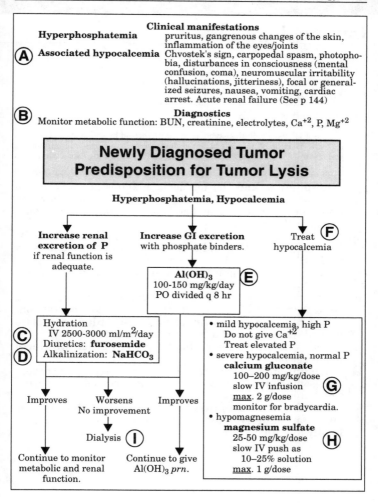

Clinical manifestations

(A) **Hyperphosphatemia** — pruritus, gangrenous changes of the skin, inflammation of the eyes/joints

Associated hypocalcemia — Chvostek's sign, carpopedal spasm, photophobia, disturbances in consciousness (mental confusion, coma), neuromuscular irritability (hallucinations, jitteriness), focal or generalized seizures, nausea, vomiting, cardiac arrest. Acute renal failure (See p 144)

(B) **Diagnostics**

Monitor metabolic function: BUN, creatinine, electrolytes, Ca^{+2}, P, Mg^{+2}

Newly Diagnosed Tumor Predisposition for Tumor Lysis

Hyperphosphatemia, Hypocalcemia

Increase renal excretion of P if renal function is adequate.

Increase GI excretion with phosphate binders.

Treat **(F)** hypocalcemia

$Al(OH)_3$ **(E)**
100-150 mg/kg/day
PO divided q 8 hr

(C) Hydration
IV 2500-3000 ml/m^2/day
(D) Diuretics: **furosemide**
Alkalinization: **NaHCO_3**

- mild hypocalcemia, high P
  Do not give Ca^{+2}
  Treat elevated P
- severe hypocalcemia, normal P
  calcium gluconate
  100–200 mg/kg/dose
  slow IV infusion **(G)**
  max. 2 g/dose
  monitor for bradycardia.
- hypomagnesemia
  magnesium sulfate
  25-50 mg/kg/dose **(H)**
  slow IV push as
  10–25% solution
  max. 1 g/dose

Improves   Worsens   Improves
            No improvement

            Dialysis **(I)**

Continue to monitor metabolic and renal function.

Continue to give $Al(OH)_3$ *prn.*

Immunology

Anaphylaxis

Kushal Vinod Raghubir

> Anaphylaxis is a clinical syndrome characterized by the acute systemic reaction of multiple organ systems to an IgE-mediated immunologic release in a previously sensitized individual. Clinical spectrum varies from mild to fatal disease.

(A) Respiratory and dermatologic manifestations are the most common clinical features of anaphylaxis. However, even mild symptoms may be warning signs of a more ominous life-threatening process.

(B) If a local antigenic area is present (e.g., IM injection, IV, bee sting), split dose and administer half the dose directly in the SC tissues of the antigenic area.

(C) Relative contraindication: ventricular tachydysrhythmias, hypertension

(D) Ensure the availability of resuscitation equipment, because diphenhydramine can cause respiratory depression.

(E) Use **racemic epinephrine or L-epinephrine**. Ensure that the administered dose is appropriate for weight.

(F) Follow the hospital protocol for continuous **albuterol** nebulization.

(G) **Theophylline** dose varies with age. See p 176 for dose.

(H) In some cases of anaphylaxis, patients can develop acute renal failure (see p 144).

(I) Use the dose of **epinephrine** as part of the SC dose given for mild symptoms, i.e., split dose and give part locally in antigenic area.

Clinical manifestations

HEENT	periorbital and perioral swelling, angioedema, injected conjunctiva, lacrimation
GI	dysphagia, crampy abdominal pain, nausea/vomiting
CNS	apprehension, sense of doom, headache, confusion
HEME	DIC
SKIN	pruritus, tingling, warmth, flushing, hives, urticaria

Patient with Anaphylaxis

➤ **Ensure ABCs.**

(A) MILD — MODERATE ☆ — SEVERE ☆

MILD

urticaria, conjunctivitis, rhinitis, mild bronchospasm

epinephrine (B)
0.01 ml/kg **SC (1:1000)**
repeat q 15 min prn.

diphenhydramine (D)
1-2 mg/kg **PO/IM**
repeat q 4-6 hr prn.

MODERATE

generalized urticaria, angioedema, stridor

epinephrine
0.01 ml/kg **IM (1:1000)**
repeat prn.

diphenhydramine
1-2 mg/kg **IV**
repeat q 4-6 hr prn.

SEVERE

stridor, respiratory failure, shock

epinephrine (C)
0.1 ml/kg IV 1:10,000)
repeat q 3-5 min prn.
• Administer succeeding doses slowly.
• If NO response start infusion at
  0.1 µg/kg/min, increase by
  0.1 µg/kg/min q min to max. of
  1.5 µg/kg/min.

methylprednisolone
2 mg/kg IV then 1 mg/kg q 6 hr

diphenhydramine
1-2 mg/kg slow IV
repeat q 4-6 hr prn.

Ensure ABCs, continue to assess. ◀── ✳(Continued on p 78)

RESPIRATORY STATUS

CARDIOVASCULAR STATUS

LARYNGEAL EDEMA
• prepare to intubate.
• hyperextend neck, jaw thrust, chin lift.
• naso/oropharyngeal airway **(E)**
racemic epinephrine by aerosol
0.5 ml of 2.25% solution with
3 ml 0.9 NS q 5 min prn
L-epinephrine (1:1000) by aerosol 3-5 ml
of undiluted solution q 5 min prn

methylprednisolone (F)
2 mg/kg IV then 1 mg/kg q 6 hr

BRONCHOSPASM
albuterol 0.3-0.5 ml/3 ml 0.9NS by aerosol, repeat prn or use continuous aerosol
0.15-0.45 mg/kg/hr max. 15 mg/hr
methylprednisolone (G)
2 mg/kg IV then 1 mg/kg q 6 hr
aminophylline 6 mg/kg loading dose IV
then continuous **theophylline** infusion
atropine 0.5 mg in 2.5 ml 0.9 NS by
aerosol prn

SHOCK (See p 28)
• Trendelenburg, if possible **(H)**
• bolus 20 ml/kg 0.9 NS, repeat prn.
• monitor urine output.
• vasopressors
  dopamine   10 - 20 µg/kg/min
  epinephrine see above dose.
methylprednisolone
2 mg/kg IV then 1 mg/kg q 6 hr

DYSRHYTHMIAS (See p 16)
lidocaine bolus 1 mg/kg IV then
20-50 µg/kg/min, cardioversion if
necessary.

☆ Notify Senior Resident, ICU. ☎ _____ ☎ _____

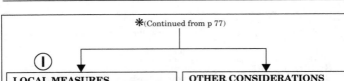

✳(Continued from p 77)

LOCAL MEASURES

When antigenic stimulant is located in extremity, e.g., bee sting, parenteral drug administration

- remove source of stimulant (IV medication, blood product).
- tourniquet proximal to antigenic site
  apply loosely, remove every 10 min. *Remember to remove tourniquet once patient is stable.*
- place extremity in dependent position.
- local ice application q 15-30 min
- local infiltration of **epinephrine** (1:10,000) 0.1–0.2 ml SC
- bee sting: remove by forceps or flicking. Do not squeeze soft tissue.

OTHER CONSIDERATIONS

- **activated charcoal** for ingested antigen 1 g/kg PO/NGT in **70% sorbitol** as initial dose
- **ranitidine** 1 mg/kg IV q 6 hr for persistent anaphylaxis
- **glucagon** 1 mg IV q 5 min prn for anaphylaxis resistant to epinephrine, specifically in patients receiving β–blocking agents

Table 7-1. ETIOLOGY: ANAPHYLAXIS (partial list)

Antibiotics	amphotericin B, cephalosporins, ketoconazole, neomycin, penicillin, sulfonamides, vancomycin
Food	bananas, beets, chocolate, citrus, egg white, fish, grains, legumes, mango, milk, nuts, preservatives, sunflower seeds
Plasma Products	whole blood, plasma, immunoglobulins, cryoprecipitate
Foreign Proteins	ACTH, antilymphocyte globulin (OKT3), chymopapain, chymotrypsin, equine antivenom, equine tetanus antitoxin, insulin, protamine, streptokinase, vasopressin

Notes

HIV ⊕ Patient with Fever

Silvia Operti-Considine

(A)   HIV ⊕ children are more likely than adults to suffer frequent severe infections because of a lack of prior immunity to the organisms.

Most common pathogens are *Streptococcus pneumoniae*, *Hemophilus influenza*, other gram-negative and staphylococcal infections. Opportunistic infections are less common than in adults.

(B)   Table 7-2.   **AGE-RELATED CHANGES OF LYMPHOCYTE PHENOTYPES OF HEALTHY CHILDREN**

	1-6 mos	7-12 mos	13-23 mos	2-6 yr	6 yr to adult
Absolute CD_4 count	3211	3128	2601	1688	1027
Percentage CD_4	51.6	47.9	45.8	42.1	50.9

Ped Res 27(abstr 916) April 1990. With permission.

(C)   In acute diarrhea, suspect a bacterial etiology if there are ≥ 5 WBC/hpf in stools, and if there is no history of prior vomiting. However, if acute diarrhea is preceded by vomiting, and there are < 5 WBC/hpf with no blood or mucus in the stools, suspect a viral etiology, e.g., Rotavirus, Cytomegalovirus, Norwalk agent.

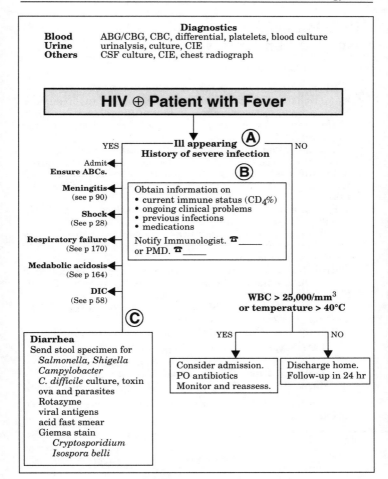

Diagnostics
Blood   ABG/CBG, CBC, differential, platelets, blood culture
Urine   urinalysis, culture, CIE
Others CSF culture, CIE, chest radiograph

HIV ⊕ Patient with Fever

Ill appearing Ⓐ
History of severe infection

YES ◄   ► NO

Admit ◄
Ensure ABCs.

Meningitis ◄
(see p 90)

Shock ◄
(See p 28)

Respiratory failure ◄
(See p 170)

Medabolic acidosis ◄
(See p 164)

DIC ◄
(See p 58)

Ⓑ
Obtain information on
• current immune status (CD$_4$%)
• ongoing clinical problems
• previous infections
• medications

Notify Immunologist. ☎ _____
or PMD. ☎ _____

WBC > 25,000/mm^3
or temperature > 40°C

YES   NO

Consider admission.   Discharge home.
PO antibiotics   Follow-up in 24 hr
Monitor and reassess.

Ⓒ

Diarrhea
Send stool specimen for
Salmonella, Shigella
Campylobacter
C. difficile culture, toxin
ova and parasites
Rotazyme
viral antigens
acid fast smear
Giemsa stain
   Cryptosporidium
   Isospora belli

HIV ⊕ Patient with Suspected Lung Involvement

Silvia Operti-Considine

(A)   Blood cultures are positive in 33% of infections of bacterial etiology. The most common pathogens involved are: *Streptococcus pneumoniae, Hemophilus influenza, Klebsiella* spp., *Staphylococcus aureus,* and *Pseudomonas aeruginosa.*

(B)   The most common opportunistic infection and the most common cause of respiratory infections in HIV ⊕ children is Pneumocystis carinii. The median age of occurrence is 5 months, and the first episode is associated with 60% mortality.

HIV ⊕ children may have normal CD4 counts and still develop *P carinii* pneumonia (PCP).

HIV ⊕ children with tachypnea and hypoxia, and a normal chest radiograph should be suspected of having PCP until proven otherwise.

Bronchoalveolar lavage (BAL) is needed to establish a definitive diagnosis. The yield remains high even 4-5 days after initiation of antimicrobial treatment.

A relapse rate of 25-85% is not uncommon in the first 12 months after completion of therapy.

Prophylaxis with one of the following is recommended:

TMP/SMZ   150 mg/750 mg/m^2/day PO qd or BID
                 for 3 consecutive days per week; or
pentamidine 4 mg/kg/dose IV q 2-4 weeks; or
dapsone   6 mg/kg/dose PO (max. 200 mg) q week

Respiratory isolation is not necessary, but protective isolation should be considered.

Age	CD4+ ≥ 20%, or unknown, with CD4+ count (cells/mm^3) of: 200 300 500 600 750 1000 1500 2000			CD4+ <20% with any CD4+ count
1-11 mos	Start PCP prophylaxis	A	B	Start PCP P R O P H Y L A X I S
12-23 mos	Start PCP prophylaxis	A	B	
24 mos-5 yr	Start PCP prophylaxis	A	B C	
≥ 6 yr	Start PCP prophylaxis	A B	C	

Figure 7-1.   Recommendations for initiation of PCP prophylaxis for children ≥ 1 mo old who are a) HIV infected, b) HIV seropositive, or c) < 12 months old and born to an HIV-infected mother

A: No prophylaxis is recommended at this time; recheck CD$_{4+}$ count in 1 month.

B: No prophylaxis is recommended at this time; recheck CD$_{4+}$ count at least every 3-4 months

C: No prophylaxis is recommended at this time; recheck CD$_{4+}$ count at least every 6 months

MMWR Vol. 40 (RR2), March 15, 1991. With permission.

✳(Continued on p 84)

Clinical manifestations

GENERAL fever
HEENT   parotitis, lymphadenopathy
RESP   hypoxia, acute tachypnea, rales, wheezing, retractions, acute/
          progressive/chronic cough
GI   hepatosplenomegaly
EXT   digital clubbing

Diagnostics

ABG/CBG, CBC, differential, platelets, LDH, blood culture (bacterial, fungal, viral, mycobacterial), urinalysis with culture, PPD with control, chest radiograph

HIV ⊕ Patient with Suspected Lung Involvement

Ensure ABCs. ◄————► Notify Senior Resident. ☎_____

O₂, pulse oximetry ◄————► Notify Immunologist. ☎_____

Clinical presentation

Acute tachypnea, hypoxia, rales, wheezing or retractions, acute non-productive cough	Progressive or chronic cough, bronchospasm, progressive hypoxia, digital clubbing; lympadenopathy, parotitis, hepatosplenomegaly

Chest radiograph findings

LOBAR INFILTRATE	**NORMAL OR DIFFUSE INTERSTITIAL INFILTRATE**	**INTERSTITIAL NODULAR PATTERN**	**Normal or mediastinal lymphadenopathy, lobar atelectasis, infiltrates/pleural effusion**
LDH normal	LDH > 500 IU/L	LDH normal	LDH normal PPD ⊕ or anergic state
Consider bacterial etiology **(A)**	Consider PCP. **(B)**	Consider LIP **(D)**	Consider mycobacteria. **(E)**
cefuroxime or **ceftazidime** if patient is in shock or has a history of *Pseudomonas* infection Consider BAL.	**TMP/SMZ** 　TMP 20 mg/kg/24 hr IV/PO divided q 6-8 hr **pentamidine** 　4 mg/kg/24 hr IV 　x 12-14 days In patients older than 13 yr who have moderate to severe PCP, consider steroids. **(C)**	O₂ as needed **prednisone** 　1-2 mg/kg/day for 1-4 weeks	**isoniazid** 　10-20 mg/kg/day PO, 　*plus* **rifampin** 　10-20 mg/kg/day PO Consider BAL, gastric aspirate or bone marrow aspirate for AFB staining and cultures to confirm diagnosis.

✳(Continued on p 84)

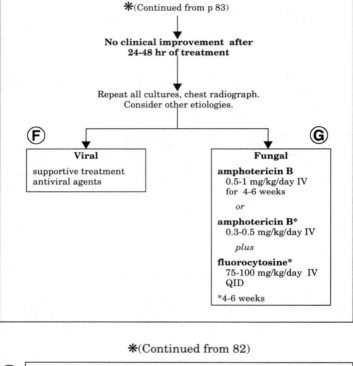

✱(Continued from p 83)

**No clinical improvement after
24-48 hr of treatment**

Repeat all cultures, chest radiograph.
Consider other etiologies.

F

Viral

supportive treatment
antiviral agents

G

Fungal

amphotericin B
0.5-1 mg/kg/day IV
for 4-6 weeks

or

amphotericin B*
0.3-0.5 mg/kg/day IV

plus

fluorocytosine*
75-100 mg/kg/day IV
QID

*4-6 weeks

✱(Continued from 82)

C

Recommendations for use of corticosteroids in treatment of acute PCP		
Indication		PaO_2 < 70 mmHg in room air or A_{-a} gradient > 35 mmHg at the time therapy is initiated
Dose	**prednisone**	40 mg PO BID x 5 days, then
		20 mg PO BID x 5 days, then
		20 mg PO qd until end of antimicrobial therapy
Note: therapy must be started within the first 72 hours of initiating antimicrobial therapy.		

AIDS Etiology, Diagnosis, Treatment and Prevention. DeVita VT, Hellman S, Rosenberg SA (eds). Philadelphia: JB Lippincott Co, 1988, p 161. With permission.

D LIP is the most common respiratory complication in HIV ⊕ patients. This may lead to chronic progressive hypoxia with bronchospasm and digital clubbing, and can sometimes be associated with hepatosplenomegaly, parotitis, and generalized lymphadenopathy. The diagnosis of LIP is based on the finding of diffuse, interstitial nodular pattern on chest radiograph, which persists for more than 2 mos in the absence of another documented cause. The definitive diagnosis is made by the presence of intraparenchymal nodular reactive hyperplasia in histologic examination of lung tissue.

(E) In infections with *Mycobacterium tuberculosis*, it is important to send BAL or biopsy specimens for susceptibility testing. If the isolated organism is resistant to isoniazid, **rifampin** and **pyrazinamide** should be added. Extrapulmonary tuberculosis is associated with 10-20% resistance to isoniazid, therefore, the addition of **pyrazinamide** 30 mg/kg/day PO is recommended.

Infections with *Mycobacterium avium-intracellulare* generally present with disseminated disease and are associated with very poor outcomes. So far, all therapeutic regimens have been unsuccessful. The median time of survival is approximately 4-5 mos.

(F) More than 2/3 of patients with measles develop disseminated disease with giant cell pneumonia. If suspected, administer **acyclovir** 1500 mg/m^2/day IV given over 1 hour TID x 7 days.

- herpes simplex infections: **acyclovir** 750 mg/m^2/day IV given over 1 hr TID x 7 days
- cytomegalovirus infections: **gancyclovir** 7.5-15 mg/kg/day IV BID
- influenza A: **amantadine** 4-6 mg/kg/day PO within 24-48 hours of appearance of symptoms until 48 hours after resolution of symptoms

(G) The most common fungal pathogens include: *Histoplasma capsulatum, Cryptococcus neoformans, Coccidioides immitis, Candida* spp. Patients on **amphotericin B** need the following determinations once a week: CBC, differential, electrolytes, BUN, creatinine, Ca^{+2}, Mg^{+2}, P, LFTs. Side effects include renal toxicity, hyperkalemia, chills and fever, bone marrow dysfunction, hypotension. With the use of **fluorocytosine**, monitor CBC, differential, platelets, creatinine, and serum drug levels. Side effects include renal and bone marrow dysfunction.

Acute Transfusion Reaction

Kushal Vinod Raghubir

> An untoward effect that results from the administration of a blood product

(A) Monitor for fluid overload.

(B) Major transfusion reactions are secondary to acute hemolysis caused by the presence of preformed recipient antibodies reacting with antigen in transfused product.

(C) Minor transfusion reactions are caused by IgA sensitization in an IgA-deficient individual.

(D) Consider other causes of fever such as sepsis, thrombophlebitis, etc.

(E) If the patient requires blood in an emergency, use washed, leukocyte-poor (preferably, HLA-compatible) blood with close monitoring of all vital signs.

(F) With the appropriate use of fluids and diuretics, and if the patient is not oliguric, **renal failure** may be averted in the early phase (See p 144).

(G) Samples to be sent to lab: donor blood (from blood bag), prereaction recipient blood (in blood bank), postreaction recipient blood, posttransfusion urine

Clinical manifestations

GENERAL	fever (≥ 1-2° rise), chills, muscle pain, chest pain, headache, local warmth at site of infusion or along vein
CVS	tachy/bradycardia, hypo/hypertension, flushing/cyanosis
RESP	tachypnea, dyspnea, cough, wheeze
GI	nausea, vomiting, abdominal cramping, and pain
RENAL	oliguria, anuria, hemoglobinuria
CNS	apprehension, sense of doom, tingling, numbness
HEME	oozing at injection/IV sites
SKIN/MUCOSA	rashes, hives, pruritus

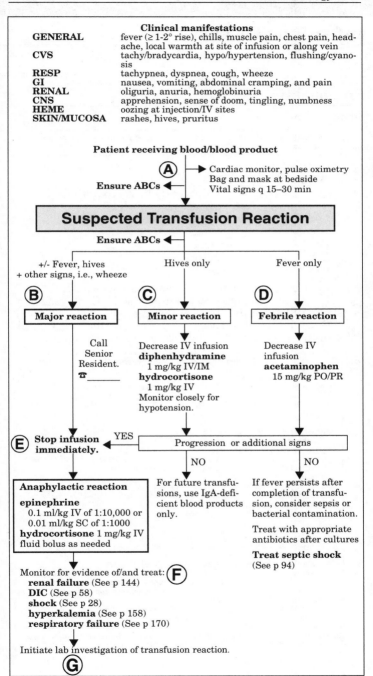

Patient receiving blood/blood product

(A) → Cardiac monitor, pulse oximetry
Bag and mask at bedside
Vital signs q 15–30 min

Ensure ABCs ←

Suspected Transfusion Reaction

Ensure ABCs ←

+/- Fever, hives
+ other signs, i.e., wheeze

Hives only

Fever only

(B) **Major reaction**

(C) **Minor reaction**

(D) **Febrile reaction**

Call
Senior
Resident.
☎_____

Decrease IV infusion
diphenhydramine
1 mg/kg IV/IM
hydrocortisone
1 mg/kg IV
Monitor closely for
hypotension.

Decrease IV
infusion
acetaminophen
15 mg/kg PO/PR

**(E) Stop infusion
immediately.** ← YES — Progression or additional signs

NO   NO

Anaphylactic reaction

epinephrine
0.1 ml/kg IV of 1:10,000 or
0.01 ml/kg SC of 1:1000
hydrocortisone 1 mg/kg IV
fluid bolus as needed

For future transfusions, use IgA-deficient blood products
only.

If fever persists after
completion of transfusion, consider sepsis or
bacterial contamination.

Treat with appropriate
antibiotics after cultures

Treat septic shock
(See p 94)

Monitor for evidence of/and treat: **(F)**
renal failure (See p 144)
DIC (See p 58)
shock (See p 28)
hyperkalemia (See p 158)
respiratory failure (See p 170)

Initiate lab investigation of transfusion reaction.

(G)

Infectious Diseases

Encephalitis

Silvia Operti-Considine

> Encephalitis is the inflammation of the brain parenchyma often associated with leptomeningeal involvement.

 CSF findings

WBC	0-500 cells/mm³
	PMNs early in the course of the disease mononuclear predominance later
Protein	normal
Glucose	normal
CIE	negative
Gram stain	negative

(B) Contraindications to lumbar puncture (see p 90)

(C) In *Herpes simplex* encephalitis, the EEG may demonstrate PLEDS or diffuse focal slowing.

(D) Once bacterial etiology and the possibility of brain abscess are excluded, antibiotics should be discontinued.

(E)

Etiologic agents in acute encephalitis		
Viruses		
Spread person to person only		
adenovirus	herpes simplex types 1 & 2	varicella-zoster
cytomegalovirus	enterovirus	reoviruses
respiratory syncytial	parainfluenza 1-3	mumps
measles	hepatitis B	human parvovirus
rubella	influenza A and B	
Spread to people by mosquitoes and ticks		
arboviruses		
Spread by warm-blooded mammals		
rabies	herpes virus simiae (herpes B)	vesicular stomatitis
encephalomyocarditis	lymphocytic choriomeningitis	
Bacteria		
Hemophilus influenza, Neiseria meningitidis, streptoccus pneumoniae, Mycobacterium tuberculosis, and other bacterial meningitides often have an encephalitic component		
Brucella spp.	Actinomycosis and Nocardia	Cat scratch disease
Other		
Chlamydia psittaci, Chlamydia pneumoniae		
rickettsial infections:	Rocky Mountain spotted fever, ehrlichiosis, Q fever, and typhus	
Mycoplasma infections:	*M. pneumoniae* and *M. hominis*	
fungal:	*C. immitis, C. neoformans*, and other fungal meningitides often have an encephalitic component.	
protozoal:	*Plasmodium* spp., *Trypanosoma* spp., *Naegleria* spp., *Acanthamoeba*, and *T. gondii*	
helminths:	trichinosis, schistosomiasis, *Strongyloides stercoralis*	
drugs:	trimethoprim	

Adapted from Feigin RD, Cherry JD. *Textbook of Pediatric Infectious Diseases*, 3rd ed, Philadelphia: WB Saunders Co, 1992, p 446. With permission.

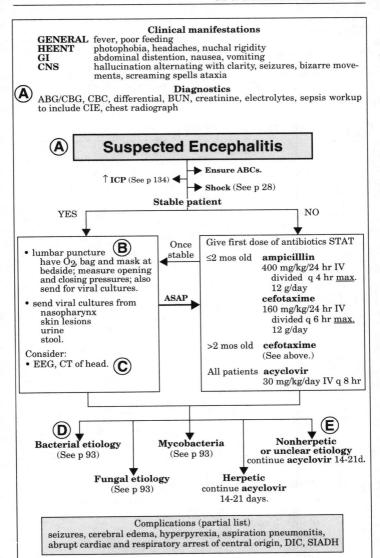

Clinical manifestations

GENERAL fever, poor feeding
HEENT photophobia, headaches, nuchal rigidity
GI abdominal distention, nausea, vomiting
CNS hallucination alternating with clarity, seizures, bizarre movements, screaming spells ataxia

(A)
Diagnostics
ABG/CBG, CBC, differential, BUN, creatinine, electrolytes, sepsis workup to include CIE, chest radiograph

(A) **Suspected Encephalitis**

↑ **ICP** (See p 134) ← ► **Ensure ABCs.**
► **Shock** (See p 28)

Stable patient

YES   NO

(B)
• lumbar puncture have O₂, bag and mask at bedside; measure opening and closing pressures; also send for viral cultures.

• send viral cultures from
  nasopharynx
  skin lesions
  urine
  stool.

Consider:
• EEG, CT of head. (C)

Once stable →

ASAP →

Give first dose of antibiotics STAT

≤2 mos old   **ampicilllin**
400 mg/kg/24 hr IV
divided q 4 hr <u>max.</u>
12 g/day
cefotaxime
160 mg/kg/24 hr IV
divided q 6 hr <u>max.</u>
12 g/day

>2 mos old   **cefotaxime**
(See above.)

All patients   **acyclovir**
30 mg/kg/day IV q 8 hr

(D)
Bacterial etiology
(See p 93)

Mycobacteria
(See p 93)

Fungal etiology
(See p 93)

(E)
Nonherpetic or unclear etiology
continue **acyclovir** 14-21d.

Herpetic
continue **acyclovir**
14-21 days.

Complications (partial list)
seizures, cerebral edema, hyperpyrexia, aspiration pneumonitis, abrupt cardiac and respiratory arrest of central origin, DIC, SIADH

Meningitis

Silvia Operti-Considine

> Infection of subarachnoid space which usually remains localized to the area in which CSF circulates. May have a rapid course which can be fatal. A high index of suspicion is needed.

(A) **Table 8-1. Typical CSF findings**

	Neonates	Infant/child	Bacterial	Partially treated	TB	Viral	Fungal
WBC/ mm^3	<30	<10	>500 (may be >60,000)	200-500	50-500	10-1000	25-500
cell type	lympho-cytes	lympho-cytes	mostly neutro-phils	lympho-cytes	lympho-cytes	*early* neutro-phils *late* lympho-cytes	lympho-cytes
glucose mg/dL	<60	> 40	<40	<40	<40	> 40	< 40
protein mg/dL	<170	10-40	>100	<40	50-500	< 100	25-500
Gram stain	negative	negative	**positive**	negative	**rarely AFB positive**	negative	**India ink positive**
culture	negative	negative	**positive**	negative	**posi-tive for AFB±**	negative	**positive (fungal)**
CIE	negative	negative	**positive**	**positive**	negative	negative	negative

(B) **Contraindications to lumbar puncture:**
   increased ICP from a space-occupying lesion, especially brain abscess
   hemophiliacs
   cardiorespiratory instability
   severe thrombocytopenia ≤ 50,000/mm^3
   DIC
   presence of infection over puncture site

✳(Continued on p 92)

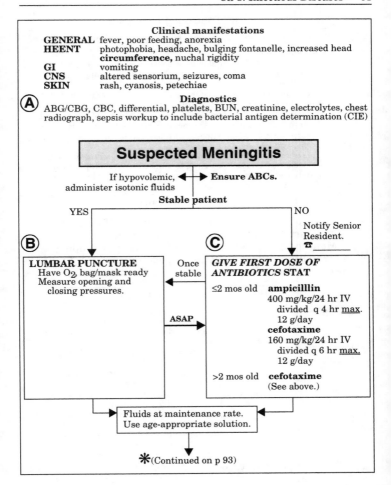

Clinical manifestations

GENERAL fever, poor feeding, anorexia
HEENT photophobia, headache, bulging fontanelle, increased head **circumference,** nuchal rigidity
GI vomiting
CNS altered sensorium, seizures, coma
SKIN rash, cyanosis, petechiae

(A) **Diagnostics**
ABG/CBG, CBC, differential, platelets, BUN, creatinine, electrolytes, chest radiograph, sepsis workup to include bacterial antigen determination (CIE)

Suspected Meningitis

If hypovolemic, ◄─► **Ensure ABCs.**
administer isotonic fluids

Stable patient

YES   NO

                                        Notify Senior
                                        Resident.
(B)   **(C)**   ☎ _____

LUMBAR PUNCTURE   Once   *GIVE FIRST DOSE OF*
Have O₂, bag/mask ready   stable   *ANTIBIOTICS* STAT
Measure opening and   ◄──
closing pressures.   ≤2 mos old **ampicilllin**
                                                400 mg/kg/24 hr IV
                          ASAP   divided q 4 hr <u>max.</u>
                          ──►   12 g/day
                                                cefotaxime
                                                160 mg/kg/24 hr IV
                                                  divided q 6 hr <u>max.</u>
                                                12 g/day

                                    >2 mos old **cefotaxime**
                                                (See above.)

        Fluids at maintenance rate.
        Use age-appropriate solution.

        ✳(Continued on p 93)

✳(Continued from p 90)

Ⓒ Dexamethasone therapy for bacterial meningitis in infants and children:

Recommendations
1. Dexamethasone therapy should be considered when bacterial meningitis in infants and children 6 weeks and older is diagnosed or strongly suspected.
2. Dexamethasone is recommended for treatment of infants and children with *H. influenza* meningitis.
3. Dexamethasone should be considered for treatment of infants and children with pneumococcal or meningococcal meningitis. However, its efficacy for these infections is unproven, and some experts do not recommend its use.
4. The recommended dexamethasone regimen is 0.6 mg/kg/day in four divided doses, given IV x 4 days. Dexamethasone therapy should be initiated as early as possible. If started more than 12 hrs after start of IV antibiotics, it is unlikely to be effective.

Adapted from the 1994 Red Book. With permission.

Ⓓ Aseptic meningitis follows a benign, self-limited course from which 95% of children recover completely.

Ⓔ Meningitis following trauma is usually secondary to *S. pneumoniae*; following neurosurgical procedures, *Staphylococcus epidermidis*.

Recommended rifampin prophylaxis	
Haemophilus influenza.	1. Households in which contact is < 48 months of age. Index patient should be given first dose just before discharge from hospital.
	2. For daycare, nursery, school and hospital contacts: See **Red Book**.
	3. Dose: **rifampin** 20 mg/kg PO (max. 600 mg/dose) daily x 4 days
Neisseria meningitidis.	1. Household, daycare, nursery, school and hospital contacts should start chemoprophylaxis ASAP. See **Red Book**.
	2. Dose: **rifampin** 20 mg/kg divided q 12 hr PO (max. 600 mg/dose) x 4 doses, i.e., 2 days. No age restriction.

Ⓕ It is important to detect fungal causes of meningitis, because therapy with **amphotericin B** or other antifungal drugs can be life-saving.

Send CSF for fungal smears. Consider serologic and antigen studies for fungi.

During the course of amphotericin B therapy, monitor BUN, creatinine, electrolytes, Ca^{+2}, Mg^{+2}, P, LFTs.

Ⓖ Obstructive hydrocephalus is extremely common in TB meningitis. Emergent neurosurgical intervention is necessary. Prognosis for survival and neurologic recovery is enhanced by early treatment.

Ⓗ *Early complications:* loss of temperature control, focal neurologic signs, brain abscess

Late complications (few days to weeks): subdural effusions, hydrocephalus, hearing loss. If fever persists > 7 days, consider subdural effusion, drug fever, phlebitis, arthritis, unrelated infections

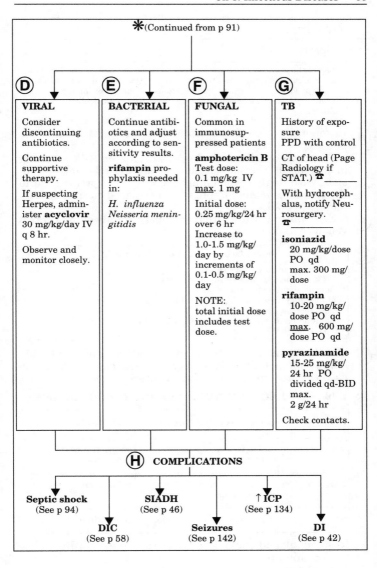

✳(Continued from p 91)

Ⓓ VIRAL

Consider discontinuing antibiotics.

Continue supportive therapy.

If suspecting Herpes, administer **acyclovir** 30 mg/kg/day IV q 8 hr.

Observe and monitor closely.

Ⓔ BACTERIAL

Continue antibiotics and adjust according to sensitivity results.

rifampin prophylaxis needed in:

H. influenza
Neisseria meningitidis

Ⓕ FUNGAL

Common in immunosuppressed patients

amphotericin B
Test dose:
0.1 mg/kg IV
max. 1 mg

Initial dose:
0.25 mg/kg/24 hr over 6 hr
Increase to 1.0-1.5 mg/kg/day by increments of 0.1-0.5 mg/kg/day

NOTE: total initial dose includes test dose.

Ⓖ TB

History of exposure
PPD with control

CT of head (Page Radiology if STAT.) ☎_____

With hydrocephalus, notify Neurosurgery.
☎_____

isoniazid
20 mg/kg/dose PO qd
max. 300 mg/dose

rifampin
10-20 mg/kg/dose PO qd
max. 600 mg/dose PO qd

pyrazinamide
15-25 mg/kg/24 hr PO divided qd-BID
max. 2 g/24 hr

Check contacts.

Ⓗ COMPLICATIONS

Septic shock
(See p 94)

DIC
(See p 58)

SIADH
(See p 46)

Seizures
(See p 142)

↑ICP
(See p 134)

DI
(See p 42)

Septic Shock

Silvia Operti-Considine

> Septic shock results from the release of microbial toxins in the blood stream causing a SIRS manifested by fever, hypotension, tachycardia, tachypnea, and evidence of organ system dysfunction or impaired organ perfusion, e.g., encephalopathy, increased lactic acid, or renal failure.

(A) In general, patients with septic shock progress through two phases:

Warm *"hyperdynamic"* phase → decreased SVR resulting in increased cardiac output to maintain adequate perfusion. With further worsening, there is rapid progression to the cold *"hypodynamic"* phase → decreased cardiac output, increased SVR.

(B) Send blood cultures from each port of indwelling central venous catheter.

(C)
> Predisposing factors associated with septic shock
>
> Intravascular line or device
> Previous therapy with multiple antibiotics
> Splenic absence or dysfunction
> Malignancy, neutropenia, sickle cell anemia
> Immunologic disorders
> Immunocompromised: neonates, malnutrition, chemotherapy, steroids, BMT

(D) If > 50 ml/kg has been given without any noticeable improvement, CVP or PA catheter measurements should be used to guide further therapeutic interventions.

(E) Table 8-2. **RECOMMENDED ANTIMICROBIAL REGIMEN**

AGE	COMMON ORGANISMS	ANTIBIOTIC
< 8 weeks	Group B *Streptococcus*, Coliforms, *Listeria*	**ampicillin and cefotaxime**
2 months - 9 yr	*S. pneumoniae, H. influenza, N. meningitidis*	**cefotaxime**
> 9 yr	*S. pneumoniae, N. meningitidis*	**cefotaxime**

Nosocomial: add staphylococcal coverage—**oxacillin, vancomycin**
Intra-abdominal: **cefotaxime, metronidazole, gentamicin**
Immunosuppressed: anti-*Pseudomonas* **ceftazidime, tobramycin**
         antifungal **amphotericin B**
         antiviral **acyclovir**

Early eradication of septic foci is essential, e.g., may need to remove or change catheters, drain abscess (notify Surgery ☎_____).

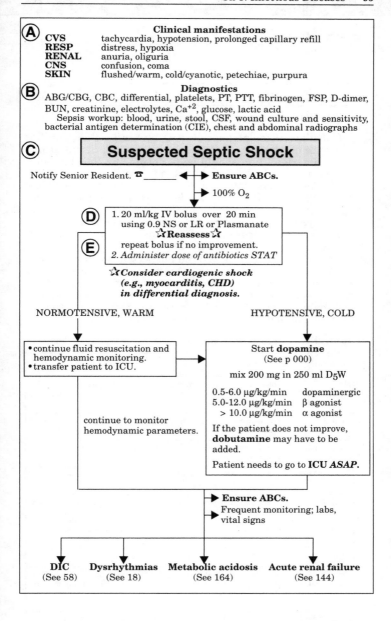

(A)

Clinical manifestations

CVS	tachycardia, hypotension, prolonged capillary refill
RESP	distress, hypoxia
RENAL	anuria, oliguria
CNS	confusion, coma
SKIN	flushed/warm, cold/cyanotic, petechiae, purpura

(B)

Diagnostics

ABG/CBG, CBC, differential, platelets, PT, PTT, fibrinogen, FSP, D-dimer, BUN, creatinine, electrolytes, Ca^{+2}, glucose, lactic acid

Sepsis workup: blood, urine, stool, CSF, wound culture and sensitivity, bacterial antigen determination (CIE), chest and abdominal radiographs

(C)

Suspected Septic Shock

Notify Senior Resident. ☎_____ ◀━━▶ **Ensure ABCs.**

▶ 100% O_2

(D)
1. 20 ml/kg IV bolus over 20 min
   using 0.9 NS or LR or Plasmanate
   ☆**Reassess**☆

(E)
   repeat bolus if no improvement.
2. *Administer dose of antibiotics STAT*

☆*Consider cardiogenic shock
(e.g., myocarditis, CHD)
in differential diagnosis.*

NORMOTENSIVE, WARM   HYPOTENSIVE, COLD

• continue fluid resuscitation and
  hemodynamic monitoring.
• transfer patient to ICU.

Start **dopamine**
(See p 000)

mix 200 mg in 250 ml D_5W

0.5-6.0 µg/kg/min	dopaminergic
5.0-12.0 µg/kg/min	β agonist
> 10.0 µg/kg/min	α agonist

continue to monitor
hemodynamic parameters.

If the patient does not improve,
dobutamine may have to be
added.

Patient needs to go to **ICU** *ASAP.*

▶ **Ensure ABCs.**
▶ Frequent monitoring; labs,
  vital signs

DIC	**Dysrhythmias**	**Metabolic acidosis**	**Acute renal failure**
(See 58)	(See 18)	(See 164)	(See 144)

Ingestions

General Poisoning

Maria Asi-Bautista

(A) Calculate osmolal gap. If >10 mOsm/L, this signifies presence of osmolal substances, e.g., alcohol. Serum osmolality determination should be performed by freezing point depression method to avoid loss of volatile osmoles. Acetaminophen, salicylate, and ethanol are common principal or coingestants. If not included in toxic screen panel, order specific levels.

A *negative* screen does *not* rule out toxic ingestion. See p 234 for list of drugs included in most toxicology panels. (Consult with your toxicology lab.)

(B) Poisoning should always be suspected when there has been an acute onset of symptoms that do not readily fit a specific disease entity. Suspect poisoning in cases of (1) head injury/trauma, (2) unexplained behavior/mental status changes, seizures, (3) dysrhythmia of unknown etiology, (4) unexplained metabolic acidosis/alkalosis.

Table 9-1. Toxic syndromes

(C)

Syndrome	Symptoms	Source (partial list)
Muscarinic (DUMBBELS)	**d**efecation, **u**rination, **m**iosis, **b**radycardia, **b**ronchorrhea, **e**mesis, **l**acrimation, **s**ecretions	acetylcholine, pilocarpine, mushrooms, betel nut, carbachol, organophosphates
Nicotinic	tachycardia, hypertension, muscle fasciculations, paralysis	insecticides (nicotinic), tobacco, black widow spider venom
Anticholinergic	dry skin, hyperthermia, thirst, dysphagia, mydriasis, tachycardia, urinary urgency and retention, delirium, hallucinations, respiratory failure	belladonna alkaloid, mushrooms, scopolamine, antihistamines, cyclic antidepressants, over-the-counter sleep medications
Sympathomimetic	CNS excitation, hypertension, convulsions, tachycardia	theophylline, caffeine, LSD, phencyclidine (PCP), cocaine, phenylpropanolamine, amphetamine
Narcotic	CNS depression, hypoventilation, hypotension, miosis	codeine, Lomotil, heroin, propoxyphene (Darvon), pentazocine (Talwin)
Narcotic withdrawal	diarrhea, mydriasis, goose bumps, tachycardia, lacrimation, yawning, cramps, hallucinations	alcohol, barbiturates, benzodiazepines, narcotics, chloral hydrate

Adapted from Ellenhorn MJ. *Medical Toxicology: Diagnosis and Treatment of Human Poisoning*, New York: Elsevier Science Publishing Company, Inc., 1988, p 26. With permission.

✳(Continued on p 99)

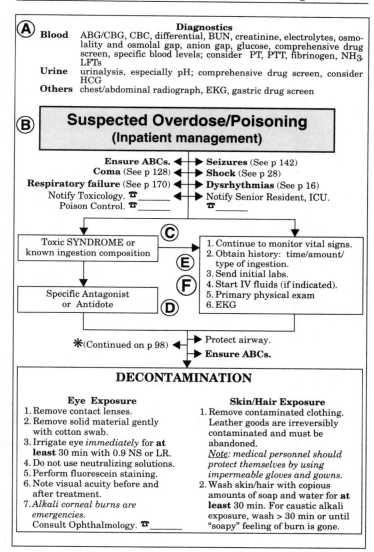

(A) **Diagnostics**

Blood ABG/CBG, CBC, differential, BUN, creatinine, electrolytes, osmolality and osmolal gap, anion gap, glucose, comprehensive drug screen, specific blood levels; consider PT, PTT, fibrinogen, NH_3, LFTs

Urine urinalysis, especially pH; comprehensive drug screen, consider HCG

Others chest/abdominal radiograph, EKG, gastric drug screen

(B) ## Suspected Overdose/Poisoning
(Inpatient management)

Ensure ABCs. ◄──► **Seizures** (See p 142)
Coma (See p 128) ◄──► **Shock** (See p 28)
Respiratory failure (See p 170) ◄──► **Dysrhythmias** (See p 16)
Notify Toxicology. ☎_____ ◄──► Notify Senior Resident, ICU.
Poison Control. ☎_____ ☎_____

Toxic SYNDROME or
known ingestion composition (C)

(E)

(F)

Specific Antagonist
or Antidote (D)

1. Continue to monitor vital signs.
2. Obtain history: time/amount/type of ingestion.
3. Send initial labs.
4. Start IV fluids (if indicated).
5. Primary physical exam
6. EKG

✱(Continued on p 98) ◄──► Protect airway.
◄──► **Ensure ABCs.**

DECONTAMINATION

Eye Exposure

1. Remove contact lenses.
2. Remove solid material gently with cotton swab.
3. Irrigate eye *immediately* for **at least** 30 min with 0.9 NS or LR.
4. Do not use neutralizing solutions.
5. Perform fluorescein staining.
6. Note visual acuity before and after treatment.
7. *Alkali corneal burns are emergencies.*
   Consult Ophthalmology. ☎_____

Skin/Hair Exposure

1. Remove contaminated clothing. Leather goods are irreversibly contaminated and must be abandoned.
   Note: medical personnel should protect themselves by using impermeable gloves and gowns.
2. Wash skin/hair with copious amounts of soap and water for **at least** 30 min. For caustic alkali exposure, wash > 30 min or until "soapy" feeling of burn is gone.

✻(Continued from p 97)

Decontamination

→ **Ensure ABCs**

Ingestions

1. INDUCE EMESIS, if patient able to protect airway

ipecac 6 mos - 1 yr	10 ml
up to 5 yr	15 ml
> 5 yr - adult	30 ml

   Repeat dose x 1 if no effect is seen within 30 min. Inspect vomitus for remnants of pills or toxic substances

   #### Contraindications
   - corrosive ingestions: strong acid/alkali
   - seizures
   - severe heart disease
   - anatomical defect that may lead to aspiration, e.g., cleft palate
   - rapid deterioration of sensorium,
   - decreasing level of consciousness
   - < 6 mos of age
   - petroleum distillate ingestion
   - absence of cough and gag reflex
   - foreign body ingestion

2. LAVAGE
   If sensorium is depressed, protect airway. Intubate if necessary, before performing lavage.
   a. position patient left side, head down
   b. **<5 yr** use 0.9 NS.
      aliquots of 50 ml. <u>min</u>. total 500 ml

      >5 yr use 0.9 NS.
      aliquots of 50-100 ml

      NOTE: tube used should be large enough to allow whole capsules and pills to be evacuated.
   c. repeat until return is clear.

   #### Contraindications
   - corrosive ingestion
   - nontoxic ingestion

3. ACTIVATED CHARCOAL

   Protect airway, then administer **activated charcoal:**
   > 1 g/kg PO (as a slurry)
   > 25-50 g in 4 oz H_2O.

   Repeat every 4 hr in cases of **phenobarbital, theophylline, cyclic antidepressant, digoxin, carbamazepine** toxicity.
   NOTE: *Some advocate giving charcoal prior to gastric lavage to prevent further absorption of toxin.*

   Drugs **not** effectively adsorbed by charcoal: **iron and other heavy metals, alcohols, organophosphates/carbamates, cyanide, hydrocarbons, caustics, and corrosives.**

4. CATHARTIC
   magnesium citrate:
   > 4 ml/kg PO/NGT
   > <u>max</u>. 300 ml/dose

   magnesium sulfate:
   > 250 mg/kg PO/NGT

   sorbitol:
   > 0.5 mg/kg PO in children
   > <u>max</u>. 50 g of 35%
   > concentration

   - may be given with first dose of charcoal.
   - do not use in trivial ingestions.
   - do not use multiple doses in children.
   - do not use sorbitol in children < 1 yr; use with caution in children < 3 yr.

   #### Contraindications
   - intestinal obstruction
   - diarrhea
   - ileus
   - renal failure (Mg^{+2})

5. WHOLE BOWEL PREPARATION
   polyethylene glycol (GoLYTELY):
   > 40 ml/kg/hr PO/NGT
   > <u>max</u>. 2 L/hr

   Especially useful for substances not adsorbed by charcoal or with ingestion of sustained release preparations

*(Continued from p 98)

(D) Table 9-2.   Common Emergency Antidotes

Poison	Antidote	Dose	Comment
Acetami- nophen	N-acetylcysteine	See p 104	
Atropine	physostigmine	0.5 mg IV over 6 sec q 20 min *prn* max. 1 mg/min	Do not use in *asthma*, dia- betes, urinary obstruction/ retention
β blocker	glucagon	100-150 μg/kg IV push then 2.5-5.0 mg/hr Taper over 5-12 hrs.	Effects of single dose observed in 5-10 min and lasts for 15-30 min
Calcium channel blocker	10%(100 mg/ml) calcium gluconate glucagon	100-200 mg/kg/dose not to exceed 2 g slow IV. Titrate to adequate response. See above dose	Monitor Ca^{+2} levels. **Contraindicated** with digitalis poisoning.
CO	O_2	100% by inhalation	t½ of COHb is 240 min in room air; if a patient is ven- tilated with 100% O_2, t½ of COHb is 60 min; in chamber at 2 atm, t½ is 25-30 min.
Iron	DFO	See p 120	
Ethylene glycol Methyl alcohol	ethyl alcohol 50% 1:1 with D_5W	See p 106	
Nitrite (methemo- globinemia)	methylene blue 1% solution (10 mg/ml)	0.2 ml/kg IV over 5 min max. dose in infants 4 mg/kg	May cause hemolysis in G6PD deficient patient.
Opiate, Darvon, Lomotil	naloxone	0.1 mg/kg/dose IV prn for reversal of respiratory depression due to opiates	max. effect 2 hr Continuous IV infusion may be needed.
Midazolam (Versed)	flumazenil (Romazicon)	0.2 mg (2 ml) IV over 30 sec, may repeat after 30 sec with 0.3 mg (3 ml). Further doses 0.5 mg over 30 sec. If no response in 5 min or max. of 5 mg, cause of sedation unlikely to be benzodiazepine.	Flumazenil is not recom- mended for cyclic antide- pressant poisoning, and if seizures and increased ICP are present.
Organo- phosphates/ carbamates	atropine, pralidoxime (2-PAM)	See p 122	

Adapted from Mofenson HC, Caraccio TR, Greensher J. Acute Poisonings. In Rakel RE (ed): *Conn's Current Therapy*, Philadelphia; WB Saunders Co, 1993, pp 1152-1161. With permission.

Ⓔ **Table 9-3. Nontoxic ingestions (partial list)**

abrasives	3% hydrogen peroxide	rubber cement
adhesives	ink	sachets
baby product cosmetics	lipstick	shampoos
ballpoint pen inks	makeup	shaving creams/lotions
bleach (less than 5%	mineral oil	soap and soap products
sodium hypochlorite)	modeling clay	suntan preparations
body conditioners	newspaper	sweetening agents
candles	perfumes	toothpaste
dehumidifying packets	petroleum jelly	watercolors
fabric softener	Play-doh	zinc oxide

Adapted from Haddad LM, Winchester JE (eds). *Clinical Management of Poisoning and Drug Overdose.* Philadelphia: WB Saunders Co., 1990. p 5. With permission.

Ⓕ Instruct family members to retrieve containers of medications or toxins whenever possible; review patient's old chart if available.

Ask about patient and family history of psychiatric problems, drug addiction, alcoholism, allergies, occupational and recreational histories, chronic diseases, asthma, sickle cell anemia. Inquire about possible medications at home, including relatives', friends' and visitors'.

All cases of *accidental* toxic ingestion need:
   1. Toxicology consult ☎_____
   2. Social Service consult ☎_____
   3. Review of old chart (if applicable)

All cases of *intentional* toxic ingestion need:
   1. All of the above
   2. Psychiatric consult ☎_____
   3. 24-hr sitter
   4. Suicide precautions

Homicide/child abuse should be suspected in infants who present with poisoning. If suspected, these children will need:
   1. All of above (except suicide precautions)
   2. Restriction of parental visits

Notes

Acetaminophen Toxicity

Maria Asi-Bautista

> Acetaminophen is a common ingredient in many over-the-counter preparations, e.g., Tylenol, Tempra, Nyquil, Contac, is also found in combination preparations, e.g., Darvocet, Tylenol with Codeine.

(A)

Phases of acetaminophen overdose			
Phase I < 24 Hours	Phase 2 24-72 Hours	Phase 3 72-96 Hours	Phase 4 1-2 Weeks
May appear normal Anorexia, nausea, vomiting	Symptoms of Phase 1 may become less prominent RUQ tenderness Abnormal LFTs	Sequelae of hepatic necrosis seen Jaundice, coagulopathy, encephalopathy, death	Hepatic regeneration Resolution of signs and symptoms

(B) Ideally, **N-acetylcysteine** and **charcoal** doses should be separated by 1-2 hours. However, in an observational study of 100 cases of acetaminophen overdose, activated charcoal had no effect on the availability of N-acetylcysteine. **If any N-acetylcysteine dose is vomited within 1 hour of administration, the dose should be repeated.**

✴(Continued on p 104)

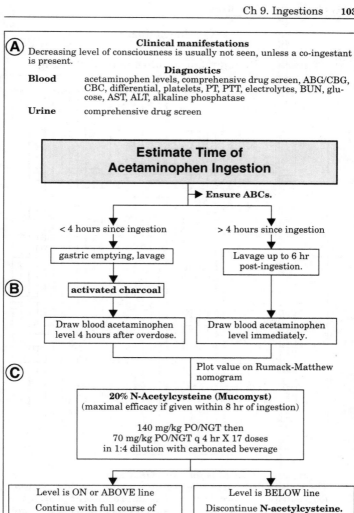

(A) **Clinical manifestations**

Decreasing level of consciousness is usually not seen, unless a co-ingestant is present.

Diagnostics

Blood   acetaminophen levels, comprehensive drug screen, ABG/CBG, CBC, differential, platelets, PT, PTT, electrolytes, BUN, glucose, AST, ALT, alkaline phosphatase

Urine   comprehensive drug screen

Estimate Time of Acetaminophen Ingestion

→ **Ensure ABCs.**

< 4 hours since ingestion

gastric emptying, lavage

> 4 hours since ingestion

Lavage up to 6 hr post-ingestion.

(B) **activated charcoal**

Draw blood acetaminophen level 4 hours after overdose.

Draw blood acetaminophen level immediately.

(C) Plot value on Rumack-Matthew nomogram

20% N-Acetylcysteine (Mucomyst)
(maximal efficacy if given within 8 hr of ingestion)

140 mg/kg PO/NGT then
70 mg/kg PO/NGT q 4 hr X 17 doses
in 1:4 dilution with carbonated beverage

Level is ON or ABOVE line

Continue with full course of **N-acetylcysteine**.

Repeat LFTs q 24 hr X 4 days while treatment in progress. If no abnormalities are found, further tests are not necessary.

Level is BELOW line

Discontinue **N-acetylcysteine.**

No further medical management needed.

Treat other medical or psychiatric problems.

INDICATIONS FOR **ORAL N-ACETYLCYSTEINE**

- serum acetaminophen level in toxic range
- estimated ingestion more than 140 mg/kg
- less than 24 hours since ingestion
- no levels available

✷(Continued from 102)

Ⓒ Rumack-Matthew Nomogram
Check units (μg/ml or μmol/L) before plotting.

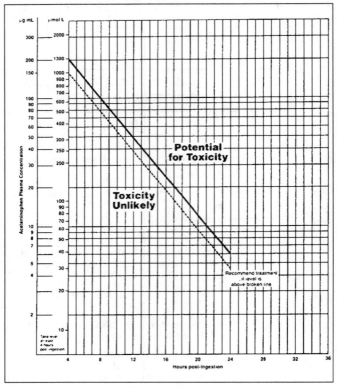

Figure 9-1. *Cautions for use of this chart*
The time coordinates refer to time post-ingestion. Serum
levels drawn before 4 hours may not represent peak levels.
The graph relates only to plasma levels following a single
acute overdose.
The broken line, which represents a 25% allowance below
the solid line, is included to allow for possible errors in acetaminophen plasma assays and estimated time from ingestion of an overdose.
Modified from Rumack BH, Matthew H. "Acetaminophen Poisoning
and Toxicity." Pediatrics 55: 871-876, 1975. With permission.

Notes

Alcohol Ingestions: Ethanol, Isopropanol, Methanol, Ethylene Glycol

Alexandre Rotta and Michelle Rotta

	Metabol-ites	High anion gap acidosis	Ketosis	CNS depres-sion	Odor or breath	Characteristic findings	Commercial uses
Ethanol	acetalde-hyde, acetic acid	+	+	+	+	alcoholic ketoacidosis not usually associated with CNS depres-sion or ethanol in blood	solvents, beverages, cologne, mouth-washes
Isopro-panol	acetone	-	+	++	+	hemorrhagic tracheobron-chitis, gastritis	rubbing alco-hol, solvents, lacquer, deicers
Methanol	formal-dehyde, formic acid (toxic)	++	-	+	-	blindness, pink edema-tous optic disc	antifreeze, solvents, gasohol, denaturant, windshield wiper fluid
Ethylene glycol	oxalic acid, glycolic acid (toxic)	++	-	+	-	renal failure, hypocalcemia, calcium oxalate crys-tals in urine	antifreeze, solvent, deic-ers, aircondi-tioning units

Modified from Goldfrank LR, Flomenbaum NE, et al. Methanol, Ethylene Gly-col, and Isopropanol. In Goldfrank's Toxicologic Emergencies, 4th ed, East Nor-walk, CT: Appleton and Lange, 1990, p 483.

Ethanol levels 100-150 mg/dL are consistent with intoxica-tion. Levels as low as 50 mg/dL can produce symptoms such as hypoglycemia, hypothermia and coma in infants and toddlers.

Potential contribution of alcohols to the osmolar gap

Substance	Gram molecular weight	mOsm/L (at 100 mg/dL)
Methanol	32	33.7
Ethanol	46	22.8
Ethylene glycol	62	19.0
Isopro-panol	60	17.6

Modified from Goldfrank LR, Flomen-baum NE, et al. *Methanol, Ethylene Glycol, and Isopropanol.* In Gold-frank's Toxicologic Emergencies, 4th ed, East Norwalk, CT: Appleton and Lange, 1990, p 483.

Estimation of blood alcohol levels

1. Calculate osmolal gap (Δ osmolality)
   Δ osmolality = measured osmolality - $\dfrac{\text{calculated osmolality}}{0.93}$
   where 0.93 is the percentage of water in serum; NOTE: measured serum osmo-lality must be determined by freezing point depression osmometer.
2. Predicted concentration (mg/dL) Serum concentration =
   $\dfrac{(\Delta \text{ osmolality})(\text{molecular weight})}{10}$
3. Example (ethylene glycol):
   Δ osmolality = 30
   Serum concentration = $\dfrac{(30)(62)}{10} = 186$ mg/dL

A normal osmolal gap **does not** rule out ingestion of a toxic alcohol.

✳(Continued on p 108)

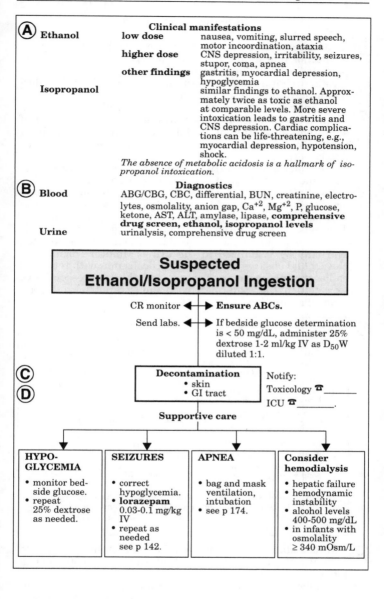

(A) Ethanol

Clinical manifestations

low dose	nausea, vomiting, slurred speech, motor incoordination, ataxia
higher dose	CNS depression, irritability, seizures, stupor, coma, apnea
other findings	gastritis, myocardial depression, hypoglycemia

Isopropanol — similar findings to ethanol. Approximately twice as toxic as ethanol at comparable levels. More severe intoxication leads to gastritis and CNS depression. Cardiac complications can be life-threatening, e.g., myocardial depression, hypotension, shock.

The absence of metabolic acidosis is a hallmark of isopropanol intoxication.

(B) Blood

Diagnostics

ABG/CBG, CBC, differential, BUN, creatinine, electrolytes, osmolality, anion gap, Ca^{+2}, Mg^{+2}, P, glucose, ketone, AST, ALT, amylase, lipase, **comprehensive drug screen, ethanol, isopropanol levels**

Urine — urinalysis, comprehensive drug screen

Suspected Ethanol/Isopropanol Ingestion

CR monitor ◄──► **Ensure ABCs.**

Send labs. ◄──► If bedside glucose determination is < 50 mg/dL, administer 25% dextrose 1-2 ml/kg IV as $D_{50}W$ diluted 1:1.

(C)
(D)

Decontamination
* skin
* GI tract

Notify:
Toxicology ☎_____
ICU ☎_____.

Supportive care

HYPO-GLYCEMIA	**SEIZURES**	**APNEA**	**Consider hemodialysis**
• monitor bedside glucose. • repeat 25% dextrose as needed.	• correct hypoglycemia. • **lorazepam** 0.03-0.1 mg/kg IV • repeat as needed see p 142.	• bag and mask ventilation, intubation • see p 174.	• hepatic failure • hemodynamic instability • alcohol levels 400-500 mg/dL • in infants with osmolality ≥ 340 mOsm/L

✱(Continued from p 106)

Ⓒ   Although activated charcoal has no role in the treatment of alcohol ingestions, it should be given to patients suspected of multiple drug or toxin ingestion.

Ⓓ   Skin decontamination is warranted due to the risk of dermal absorption and inhalation.

Ⓔ   Symptoms may not be apparent initially. There is a latent period of about 8-24 hours prior to development of symptoms in methanol, and 1-4 hours in ethylene glycol ingestions. Patients need to be monitored closely for deterioration.

With methanol ingestion, blurring of vision may lead to permanent visual loss if not managed promptly.

Ⓕ   Both methanol and ethylene glycol ingestions result in severe acidosis with a high anion gap. However, an initial normal pH does not rule out significant ingestion/toxicity. The hypocalcemia observed in ethylene glycol ingestion is due to chelation of Ca^{+2} by oxalate which is then excreted and may be visualized in the urine. Monitor serum Ca^{+2} closely and observe for signs of hypocalcemia with tetany. If radiator antifreeze was ingested, the fluorescent dye excreted in the urine can be demonstrated by a Wood's lamp examination.

Ⓖ

Calculation of ethanol infusion		
Vd:	desired serum concentration (mg/dL)	100-150 mg/dL
adult 0.6 L/kg	specific gravity of 100% ethanol	0.79
child 0.7 L/kg	10% ethanol	
	(10 ml 100% ethanol + 90 ml D_5W)	79 mg/ml

1. To calculate loading dose
   dose = (Vd)(Cp) where Cp is desired plasma concentration

   $$= \left(\frac{0.7L}{kg} \times \frac{10dL}{L} \right) \left(\frac{100mg}{dL} \right) = \left(\frac{700mg}{kg} \times \frac{1ml}{79mg} \right) = 8.86 \text{ or } 9 \text{ ml/kg}$$

2. To calculate maintenance dose
   ethanol clearance 125 mg/kg/hour

   $$dose = \left(\frac{125mg}{kg} \times \frac{1ml}{79mg} \right) = 1.58 \text{ or } 1.6 \text{ ml/kg/hr}$$

3. If IV ethanol is unavailable and patient does not have altered mental status, 20%–30% concentration (40–60 proof) may be administered through an NGT. IV ethanol solution should be started as soon as possible.

Ⓗ   If hemodialysis is instituted, the ethanol infusion should be continued at twice the usual infusion rate $\cong$ 250-350 mg/kg/hour.

Ⓘ   In laboratory animals, folic acid promotes catalase-mediated metabolism of formate to CO_2 and H_2O. Whether it has the same effects on humans is unclear.

Ⓙ   Pyridoxine and thiamine are cofactors in the metabolism of ethlylene glycol that lead to the formation of nontoxic metabolites.

(E) **Clinical manifestations**

Methanol   nausea, vomiting, abdominal pain, GI bleeding, pancre-
                   atitis, CNS depression, irritability, headache, dizziness,
                   stupor, coma, apnea. Cloudy or blurred vision is charac-
                   teristic and may lead to blindness.

Ethylene Glycol **Stage 1 (4-8 hr)**   CNS depression, lethargy, seizures,
                                          coma, tetany, persistent vomiting,
                                          cardiac dysrhythmias
                   Stage 2 (8-16 hr) coma, cardiopulmonary failure
                   Stage 3 (24-72 hr) acute tubular necrosis/renal failure

(B)(F) **Diagnostics**

Blood   ABG/CBG, CBC, differential, platelets, BUN, creatinine, electro-
           lytes, osmolality, anion gap, CA^{+2}, Mg^{+2}, P, glucose, ketone, AST,
           ALT, amylase, lipase, **comprehensive drug screen, metha-
           nol, ethylene glycol levels**

Urine   urinalysis with microscopy, occult blood, comprehensive drug
           screen

Others EKG (QTc), Wood's lamp examination of face, chest, mouth, and
           urine; stool for occult blood

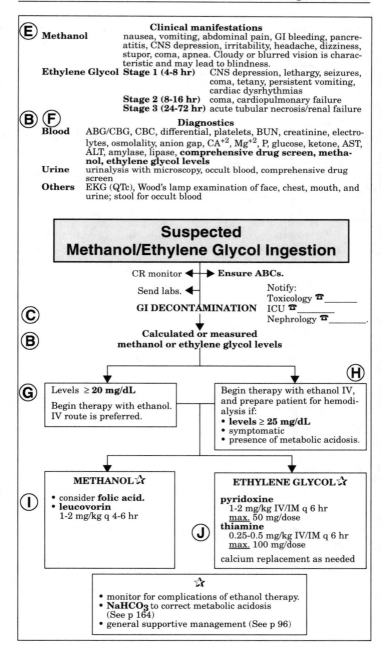

Suspected
Methanol/Ethylene Glycol Ingestion

CR monitor ←→ **Ensure ABCs.**

Send labs. ←

(C) **GI DECONTAMINATION**

Notify:
Toxicology ☎_____
ICU ☎_____
Nephrology ☎_____.

(B) **Calculated or measured
methanol or ethylene glycol levels**

(G) Levels **≥ 20 mg/dL**

Begin therapy with ethanol.
IV route is preferred.

(H) Begin therapy with ethanol IV,
and prepare patient for hemodialysis if:
• **levels ≥ 25 mg/dL**
• symptomatic
• presence of metabolic acidosis.

METHANOL ☆
• consider **folic acid.**
(I) • **leucovorin**
  1-2 mg/kg q 4-6 hr

ETHYLENE GLYCOL ☆
pyridoxine
  1-2 mg/kg IV/IM q 6 hr
  <u>max.</u> 50 mg/dose
(J) **thiamine**
  0.25-0.5 mg/kg IV/IM q 6 hr
  <u>max.</u> 100 mg/dose

calcium replacement as needed

☆
• monitor for complications of ethanol therapy.
• **NaHCO₃** to correct metabolic acidosis
  (See p 164)
• general supportive management (See p 96)

Caustic Ingestion/Exposure

Maria Asi-Bautista

> Acids and alkaline agents are caustic chemicals that can cause direct tissue damage. Alkalis cause deep penetrating liquefaction necrosis that can result in GI perforation, usually in the esophagus. Acids produce superficial coagulation necrosis with eschar formation.

(A) Patients with significant exposure to a caustic substance develop symptoms early and are usually critically ill.

*Serious esophageal injury may be present **even** in the absence of oral burns.*

A thorough examination is needed to determine the presence of (1) other areas of burns and (2) other associated injuries, e.g., if suspecting child abuse.

(B) Comprehensive drug screens need to be obtained if suicide is suspected, and in instances of multiple ingestions.

An esophagogram is not reliable and, therefore, is not indicated in the acute phase of caustic ingestions. Obtain chest radiographs to look for evidence of aspiration, pneumonitis, mediastinitis; abdominal radiographs to look for free air in the peritoneal cavity.

If a pH meter is not available, reagent strips for urinalysis may be used to determine pH.

After irrigating the eyes with sterile saline or water, test pH of the ocular cul-de-sac to ensure adequate neutralization. Normal pH of tears is 7.

(C) It is important to determine the type of caustic substance ingested (see table p 112). The following information is necessary: (1) amount/type of ingestion, (2) product concentration, and (3) time of ingestion. If possible, have a family member bring the suspected poison in its original container.

(D) Respiratory symptoms can develop following ingestion/inhalation of laundry detergents and oven cleaners (NaOH). Observe for worsening of respiratory symptoms secondary to airway obstruction.

(E) *Alkali burn to the cornea is always an emergency!* Consult Ophthalmology. ☎_____

(F) To assess extent of damage, endoscopy should be performed within 6-24 hours of ingestion, or earlier if symptomatic.

(G) If suspecting esophageal perforation, or if the patient presents with a clinical picture compatible with a surgical abdomen, DO NOT perform GI decontamination. Notify Surgery service emergently.

✳(Continued on p 112)

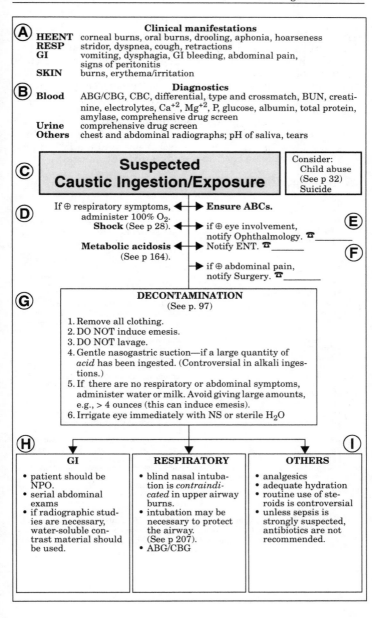

(A)

Clinical manifestations

HEENT	corneal burns, oral burns, drooling, aphonia, hoarseness
RESP	stridor, dyspnea, cough, retractions
GI	vomiting, dysphagia, GI bleeding, abdominal pain, signs of peritonitis
SKIN	burns, erythema/irritation

(B)

Diagnostics

Blood	ABG/CBG, CBC, differential, type and crossmatch, BUN, creatinine, electrolytes, Ca^{+2}, Mg^{+2}, P, glucose, albumin, total protein, amylase, comprehensive drug screen
Urine	comprehensive drug screen
Others	chest and abdominal radiographs; pH of saliva, tears

(C)

Suspected Caustic Ingestion/Exposure

Consider:
Child abuse
(See p 32)
Suicide

(D) If ⊕ respiratory symptoms, ◄──► **Ensure ABCs.**
administer 100% O_2.
Shock (See p 28). ◄──► if ⊕ eye involvement,
notify Ophthalmology. ☎_____ **(E)**

Metabolic acidosis ◄──► Notify ENT. ☎_____
(See p 164). **(F)**

──► if ⊕ abdominal pain,
notify Surgery. ☎_____

(G)

DECONTAMINATION
(See p. 97)

1. Remove all clothing.
2. DO NOT induce emesis.
3. DO NOT lavage.
4. Gentle nasogastric suction—if a large quantity of *acid* has been ingested. (Controversial in alkali ingestions.)
5. If there are no respiratory or abdominal symptoms, administer water or milk. Avoid giving large amounts, e.g., > 4 ounces (this can induce emesis).
6. Irrigate eye immediately with NS or sterile H_2O

(H) **(I)**

GI	**RESPIRATORY**	**OTHERS**
• patient should be NPO. • serial abdominal exams • if radiographic studies are necessary, water-soluble contrast material should be used.	• blind nasal intubation is *contraindicated* in upper airway burns. • intubation may be necessary to protect the airway. (See p 207). • ABG/CBG	• analgesics • adequate hydration • routine use of steroids is controversial • unless sepsis is strongly suspected, antibiotics are not recommended.

*(Continued from p 110)

(H) Caustics in liquid form (strong bases) are more commonly associated with strictures of the esophagus.

Barium swallow or esophagogram is recommended 10-20 days following injury.

(I) Corticosteroids are used for second-degree circumferential burns. For maximum efficacy, corticosteroids should be started within 48 hours of injury.

Contraindications: GI bleeding, perforation

methylprednisolone   < 2 yr old   20 mg IV q 8 hr
                         > 2 yr old   40 mg IV q 8 hr

If patient is on corticosteroids, start antibiotics.

Table 9-5.   Chemical Agents Causing Burns

Chemical agent	Commercial product
Acetic acid	Permanent wave neutralizers
Acids (tungstic, picric, tannic) (and see below)	Industrial utilization
Ammonia	Toilet bowl cleaners, metal cleaners and polishes, hairdyes and tints, antirust products, jewelry cleaners, floor strippers, glass cleaners
Batteries	Hearing aids, cameras, watches, calculators
Benzalkonium chloride	Detergents
Boric acid	Roach powders, water softener, germicides
Cantharides (Spanish fly)	Aphrodisiac (in animals), hair tonic, abortifacient
Formaldehyde (formic acid)	Deodorizing tablets, plastic menders, fumigant, embalming agent
Hydrochloric acid (muriatic acid)	Metal and toilet bowl cleaners
Hydrofluoric acid	Antirust products
Iodine	Antiseptics
Methylethyl ketone peroxide	Industrial synthetic agent
Oxalic acid	Disinfectants, household bleach, metal cleaning liquids, antirust products, furniture polish
Phenol (cresol, creosote)	Antiseptics, preservatives
Phosphoric acid	Toilet bowl cleaners
P	Matches, rodenticides, fireworks, insecticides
Potassium permanganate	Illegitimate abortifacient, medical applications (topical)
NaOH	Detergents, Clinitest tablets, washing powders, paint removers, drain cleaners and openers (Drano, Liquid-Plumr), oven cleaners
Sodium borates, carbonates, phosphates and silicates	Detergents, electric dishwasher preparations, water softeners
Sodium hypochlorite	Bleaches, cleansers
Sulfuric acid	Automobile batteries, drain cleaners
Zinc chloride	Soldering flux

From Hoffman RS, Goldfrank LR, Howland MA. Caustics and Batteries In Goldfrank, LR (ed), *Goldfrank's Toxicologic Emergencies*, 4th ed. East Norwalk, CT: Appleton and Lange, 1990, p 770. With permission.

Notes

Cyclic Antidepressant Overdose

Maria Asi-Bautista

> **Suspect** CA overdose in any patient with signs of anticholinergic poisoning, hypotension, and coma.
>
> **Indications** for CA use in children include treatment of (1) school phobia, (2) depression, (3) sleep disorders, (4) hyperkinesia, and (5) enuresis.
>
> **Commonly available preparations:**
> doxepin (Sinequan), imipramine (Tofranil), desipramine (Norpramin), amitriptyline (Elavil, Endep), nortriptyline (Pamelor)

(A) Signs and symptoms generally develop 4 hr after ingestion. Cardiovascular toxicity is the most common cause of death and usually develops within 6 hr of ingestion.

Mnemonic for anticholinergic overdose:
"**Hot** as a hare
Blind as a bat
Red as a beet
Dry as a bone
Mad as a hatter"

(B) Cyclic antidepressant levels are not useful in initial assessment. Levels are rarely available on a STAT basis. Qualitative assay is useful only in the documentation of CA ingestion.

(C) Family, social, and mental health histories may provide important clues to diagnosis. Ask for medication list of all household occupants *and* visitors.

(D) **Do not induce emesis.** Rapid neurologic deterioration is known to occur.

Gastric lavage using large bore orogastric tube may be useful if performed soon after ingestion. Sorbitol should be given with the FIRST charcoal dose.

(E) QRS > 0.10 sec predicts development of seizures and dysrhythmias and is the best indicator for severity of overdose.

(F) 95% of CA is protein-bound in serum. Acidosis increases the availability of CA by decreasing CA binding.

(G) CAs block the reuptake of norepinephrine at the neuromuscular junction. Inotropic agents such as dopamine, which in part rely on norepinephrine release from storage vesicles, may be ineffective.

(A) ANTICHOLINERGIC

Clinical manifestations

urinary retention, mydriasis, dry mouth, hypertension, fever, decreased bowel sounds

CVS   hypertension/hypotension, sinus tachycardia, ventricular tachycardia, conduction block, sudden death

CNS   seizures, coma, lethargy, disorientation, hallucinations, myoclonus

(B)   **Diagnostics**

Blood   comprehensive drug screen, ABG/CBG, CBC, differential, electrolytes, BUN, creatinine

Urine   comprehensive drug screen

Other   chest radiograph, EKG

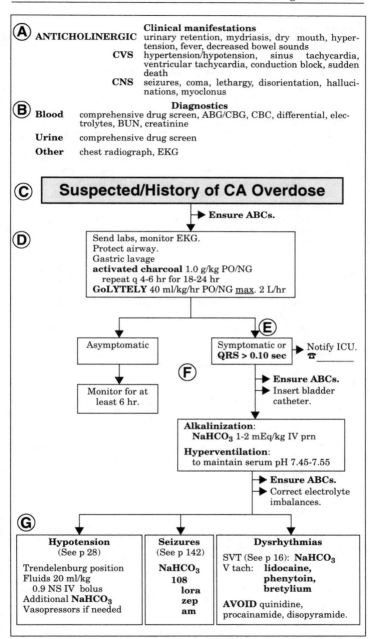

(C) Suspected/History of CA Overdose

→ **Ensure ABCs.**

(D) Send labs, monitor EKG.
Protect airway.
Gastric lavage
activated charcoal 1.0 g/kg PO/NG
repeat q 4-6 hr for 18-24 hr
GoLYTELY 40 ml/kg/hr PO/NG <u>max</u>. 2 L/hr

Asymptomatic

Monitor for at least 6 hr.

(E) Symptomatic or **QRS > 0.10 sec** → Notify ICU. ☎____

(F) → **Ensure ABCs.**
→ Insert bladder catheter.

Alkalinization:
NaHCO₃ 1-2 mEq/kg IV prn

Hyperventilation:
to maintain serum pH 7.45-7.55

→ **Ensure ABCs.**
→ Correct electrolyte imbalances.

(G)

Hypotension
(See p 28)

Trendelenburg position
Fluids 20 ml/kg
0.9 NS IV bolus
Additional **NaHCO₃**
Vasopressors if needed

Seizures
(See p 142)

NaHCO₃
108
lora
zep
am

Dysrhythmias

SVT (See p 16): **NaHCO₃**
V tach: **lidocaine,**
phenytoin,
bretylium

AVOID quinidine, procainamide, disopyramide.

Hydrocarbon Exposure

Maria Asi-Bautista

(A) Fever within 24 hours is usually related to direct tissue toxicity and not to infection.

Aspiration pneumonitis following ingestion is a common presentation. Following inhalation, cardiovascular and neurologic toxicities are major concerns, especially in cases of abuse, e.g., "huffing" or "bagging" of glue solvents, gasoline, etc.

(B) Laboratory values may be normal immediately following ingestion and need to be repeated within 48 hours.

Send for comprehensive serum and urine drug screens to determine whether other harmful toxic additives and drugs may also have been ingested.

Early chest radiograph prior to development of signs and symptoms is not predictive of the development of aspiration pneumonia.

Leukocytosis may be secondary to chemical pneumonitis.

(C) In general, risk for aspiration following ingestion is greatest with hydrocarbons with low viscosity and surface tension.

See p 118 for table of petroleum (and pine) distillates toxic to humans.

(D) Hypoglycemia and concomitant opioid abuse may complicate clinical picture.

(E)

Indications for gastric evacuation

Emesis with syrup of ipecac
  Indicated when there is:
  • toxic petroleum distillates or turpentine in *massive* quantities
  • presence of toxic additive (CHAMP)* (consider amount, type)
  • concomitant ingestion of another toxic substance for which ipecac would be indicated
  Contraindicated when there is:
  • accidental ingestion of a "pure" petroleum distillate or turpentine in a child (small quantity)
  • previous unprovoked emesis
  • presence of neurologic, respiratory, or cardiac abnormalities, or absent gag reflex (or if these signs and symptoms are expected to develop)

Gastric lavage
  Indicated when:
  • removal of liquid substance is indicated but ipecac-induced emesis is contraindicated (NG lavage acceptable)
  • an additional toxic substance was ingested for which lavage would be indicated (orogastric lavage preferable)
  • rapid onset of the toxin's activity is expected
*camphor, halogenated hydrocarbons, aromatics, metals, pesticides

---

Adapted from Goldfrank LR. *Goldfrank's Toxicologic Emergencies*, 5th ed. East Norwalk, CT: Appleton and Lange, 1994, p 1234. With permission.

✻(Continued on p 118)

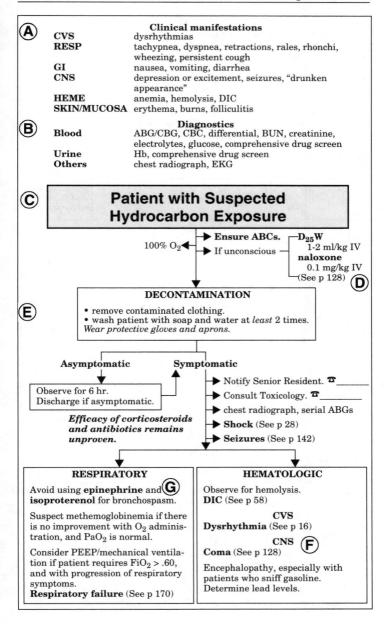

(A)

	Clinical manifestations
CVS	dysrhythmias
RESP	tachypnea, dyspnea, retractions, rales, rhonchi, wheezing, persistent cough
GI	nausea, vomiting, diarrhea
CNS	depression or excitement, seizures, "drunken appearance"
HEME	anemia, hemolysis, DIC
SKIN/MUCOSA	erythema, burns, folliculitis

(B)

	Diagnostics
Blood	ABG/CBG, CBC, differential, BUN, creatinine, electrolytes, glucose, comprehensive drug screen
Urine	Hb, comprehensive drug screen
Others	chest radiograph, EKG

(C)

Patient with Suspected Hydrocarbon Exposure

➤ **Ensure ABCs.**

100% O₂ ◄─── | If unconscious ─── **D₂₅W** 1-2 ml/kg IV
naloxone 0.1 mg/kg IV
(See p 128) **(D)**

(E)

DECONTAMINATION
• remove contaminated clothing.
• wash patient with soap and water at *least* 2 times.
Wear protective gloves and aprons.

Asymptomatic   **Symptomatic**

Observe for 6 hr.
Discharge if asymptomatic.

Efficacy of corticosteroids and antibiotics remains unproven.

➤ Notify Senior Resident. ☎ _____
➤ Consult Toxicology. ☎ _____
➤ chest radiograph, serial ABGs
➤ **Shock** (See p 28)
➤ **Seizures** (See p 142)

RESPIRATORY

Avoid using **epinephrine** and **(G) isoproterenol** for bronchospasm.

Suspect methemoglobinemia if there is no improvement with O₂ administration, and PaO₂ is normal.

Consider PEEP/mechanical ventilation if patient requires FiO₂ > .60, and with progression of respiratory symptoms.
Respiratory failure (See p 170)

HEMATOLOGIC

Observe for hemolysis.
DIC (See p 58)

CVS
Dysrhythmia (See p 16)

CNS (F)
Coma (See p 128)

Encephalopathy, especially with patients who sniff gasoline.
Determine lead levels.

✳(Continued from 116)

Table 9-6. Petroleum (and pine) distillates toxic to humans

Product	Volatility	Viscosity	Toxicity[a]		Uses
			CNS mechanism	Pulmonary aspiration	
Gases	H	L	+ (ASP)	0	Fuel
Benzine (aliphatics, trace aromatics)	H	L	+ (ASP)	0	Solvent
Aromatics, benzene, toluene, xylene	H	L	+ (INH) (ABS)	±	solvent, degreaser, Most toxic CNS depressant
Gasoline	H	L	+ (INH)	±	Fuel
Naphtha	H	L	+ (INH)	±	Lighter fuel, lacquer diluent
Mineral spirits	L	L	± (INH)	+	Solvent, degreaser
Kerosene	L	L	± (INH)	+	Lighter fluid, fuel
Light gas oil	L	L	+ (INH)	+	Diesel, home fuels
Mineral seal oil	L	L	± (INH)	+	Furniture polish
Mineral oil	L	H	0	+	Baby oil, laxative
Heavy gas oil	L	H	0	±	Motor oil, transmission fluid
Lubricants	L	H	0	0	Paraffin, wax, petroleum jelly

From Goldfrank LR, *Goldfrank's Toxicologic Emergencies*, 5th ed. East Norwalk, CT: Appleton and Lange, 1994, p 1238. With permission.

[a] Extent of Toxicity
+ = major; ± = occasional/minor; 0 = generally absent.
ASP = asphyxia; INH = inhalation.
H = high (> 100 SSU); L = low (< 60 SSU).
These products are listed in increasing order of molecular weight, number of carbons, and boiling point from gases at the lowest and lubricants the highest.

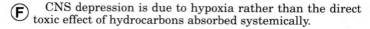

Ⓕ CNS depression is due to hypoxia rather than the direct toxic effect of hydrocarbons absorbed systemically.

Ⓖ   The myocardium develops an increased sensitivity to catecholamines that may lead to dysrhythmias.

Occasionally, hydrocarbons are used as a solvent for insecticides. Anticipate cholinergic crises secondary to organophosphate/carbamate poisoning. (See p 122)

Persistence of coughing usually signifies that aspiration has occurred.

Iron Poisoning

Maria Asi-Bautista

> Increasing incidence of toxicity is seen as a result of (1) easy availability, (2) high doses of iron in prenatal vitamins, and (3) brightly colored, sugar-coated tablets that resemble candy. Toxicity is seen with ingestions of > 60 mg/kg elemental iron, but may also be seen with doses as low as 20-60 mg/kg.

(A)

Clinical stages of iron toxicity	Elemental iron equivalents
Stage 1: *< 6 hr post-ingestion* Nausea, vomiting, severe gastroenteritis, hematemesis, hematochezia, abdominal pain, coagulopathy, lethargy	Ferrous sulfate (hydrate)20% Ferrous sulfate (dried) 37% Ferrous gluconate 12% Ferrous fumarate 33% Ferrous lactate 19% Ferrous chloride 28% Ferrous ferrocholinate 13% Ferric phosphate 37% Ferric pyrophosphate 12%
Stage 2: *latent period 6-24 hr* Deceptive improvement. Observe closely. Continue therapy.	
Stage 3: *systemic toxicity 4-40 hr* Restlessness, disorientation, lethargy, coma, convulsions, fever, shock, coagulopathy	Example: $FeSO_4$ 325 mg x 0.2 = 65 mg of elemental Fe
Stage 4: *7-10 days* Hepatic and renal failure possible	
Stage 5: *late complications, days - weeks* GI obstruction 2° to scarring and strictures (pyloric, antral, intestinal)	Ferrous oxide **does not** cause toxicity.

(B) Use heparinized tube for serum iron determinations. Levels are most useful 3-4 hr postingestion for liquids/tablets. Repeat levels 3-4 hr later (if atomic absorptive spectrophotometry available), if sustained release/enteric-coated product ingested. **Notify lab if child is on DFO, because DFO alters serum levels of iron.**

(C) Do not use activated charcoal. May use isotonic **NaHCO₃** solution for lavage. Fleets phosphosoda enema and lavage with DFO are not recommended.

(D) Use **GoLYTELY** PO or per NGT in **children** 40 ml/kg/hr; **adults** 2L/hr until rectal effluent is clear.

(E) *Yersinia enterocolitica* septicemia has been described in previously healthy children being treated for iron overdose with deferoxamine.

(F) Serum glucose > 150 mg/dL and WBC > 15,000 mm³ *suggests* SI > 300 µg/dL.

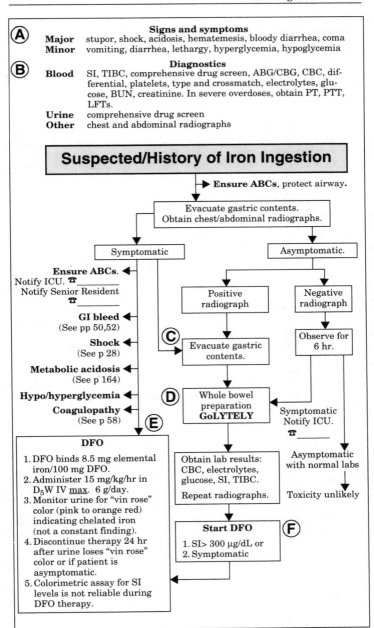

(A) **Signs and symptoms**
Major stupor, shock, acidosis, hematemesis, bloody diarrhea, coma
Minor vomiting, diarrhea, lethargy, hyperglycemia, hypoglycemia

(B) **Diagnostics**
Blood SI, TIBC, comprehensive drug screen, ABG/CBG, CBC, differential, platelets, type and crossmatch, electrolytes, glucose, BUN, creatinine. In severe overdoses, obtain PT, PTT, LFTs.
Urine comprehensive drug screen
Other chest and abdominal radiographs

Suspected/History of Iron Ingestion

➤ **Ensure ABCs**, protect airway.

Evacuate gastric contents.
Obtain chest/abdominal radiographs.

Symptomatic | Asymptomatic.

Ensure ABCs. ◄
Notify ICU. ☎_____
Notify Senior Resident
☎_____

GI bleed ◄
(See pp 50,52)

Shock ◄
(See p 28)

Metabolic acidosis ◄
(See p 164)

Hypo/hyperglycemia ◄

Coagulopathy ◄
(See p 58)

(E)

Positive radiograph | Negative radiograph

(C) Evacuate gastric contents. | Observe for 6 hr.

(D) Whole bowel preparation **GoLYTELY**

Symptomatic
Notify ICU.
☎_____

Asymptomatic with normal labs

Toxicity unlikely

DFO
1. DFO binds 8.5 mg elemental iron/100 mg DFO.
2. Administer 15 mg/kg/hr in D_5W IV <u>max</u>. 6 g/day.
3. Monitor urine for "vin rose" color (pink to orange red) indicating chelated iron (not a constant finding).
4. Discontinue therapy 24 hr after urine loses "vin rose" color or if patient is asymptomatic.
5. Colorimetric assay for SI levels is not reliable during DFO therapy.

Obtain lab results: CBC, electrolytes, glucose, SI, TIBC.

Repeat radiographs.

Start DFO **(F)**
1. SI> 300 µg/dL or
2. Symptomatic

Organophosphate/Carbamate Poisoning

Maria Asi-Bautista

> Organophosphates/carbamates are used as insecticides, miticides, and aphicides. Organophosphates/carbamates are associated with accidental and intentional ingestion in home and workplace.

(A) Organophosphates and carbamates produce identical symptomatology *except* that carbamate intoxication is usually limited to a 1- to 2-day course because the carbamate-AchE bond is easily hydrolyzed, has poor CNS penetration, and therefore has limited CNS toxicity. Absorption: transdermal (slowest), transconjunctival, across GI, GU mucosa, and through inhalation (most rapid).

Hydrocarbons are occasionally used as a vehicle for insecticides/pesticides, and toxicity secondary to hydrocarbon exposure may occur (See p 116).

(B) Hyperglycemia and glycosuria without ketosis may occur in severe poisoning.

Erythrocyte AChe and plasma chE activity should be measured to document poisoning. Follow erythrocyte AChe activity after **pralidoxime (2-PAM)** therapy. Levels are not immediately available and therefore cannot be used to guide therapy.

Plasma chE is a more sensitive indicator of exposure. Erythrocyte AChe better correlates with clinical effects.

(C) **DO NOT DELAY intervention if organophosphate poisoning is strongly suspected.**

Atropine (antimuscarinic) may also be given *via subcutaneous, intraosseous, or endotracheal* route. It has *no* effect on skeletal muscle weakness, paralysis, or actual rate of restoration of inhibited enzymes. Tachycardia is *not* a contraindication to the use of atropine. Adjust dose according to clinical effects.

Medical observation for at least 24 hours is advised if atropine has been administered.

(D) **Pralidoxime (2-PAM)** ameliorates both the muscarinic and nicotinic effects by regeneration of cholinesterases. CNS symptoms are ameliorated as well. It can be used in *both* carbamate as well as organophosphate poisoning. Although it is more effective when given in the first 24-48 hours, **patients presenting late may still benefit from this medication.** Note: rapid infusion of pralidoxime is associated with transient hypertension.

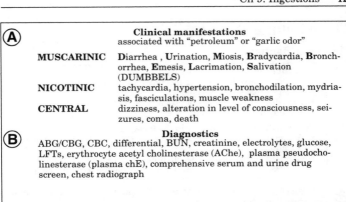

(A) **Clinical manifestations**
associated with "petroleum" or "garlic odor"

MUSCARINIC	**D**iarrhea , **U**rination, **M**iosis, **B**radycardia, **B**ronch-orrhea, **E**mesis, **L**acrimation, **S**alivation (DUMBBELS)
NICOTINIC	tachycardia, hypertension, bronchodilation, mydriasis, fasciculations, muscle weakness
CENTRAL	dizziness, alteration in level of consciousness, seizures, coma, death

(B) **Diagnostics**
ABG/CBG, CBC, differential, BUN, creatinine, electrolytes, glucose, LFTs, erythrocyte acetyl cholinesterase (AChe), plasma pseudocholinesterase (plasma chE), comprehensive serum and urine drug screen, chest radiograph

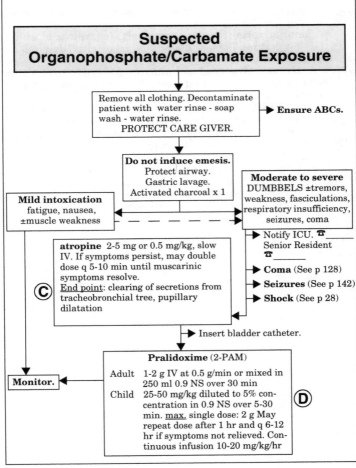

Suspected Organophosphate/Carbamate Exposure

Remove all clothing. Decontaminate patient with water rinse - soap wash - water rinse. PROTECT CARE GIVER. → **Ensure ABCs.**

Do not induce emesis.
Protect airway.
Gastric lavage.
Activated charcoal x 1

Mild intoxication
fatigue, nausea, ±muscle weakness

Moderate to severe
DUMBBELS ±tremors, weakness, fasciculations, respiratory insufficiency, seizures, coma

(C) **atropine** 2-5 mg or 0.5 mg/kg, slow IV. If symptoms persist, may double dose q 5-10 min until muscarinic symptoms resolve.
<u>End point</u>: clearing of secretions from tracheobronchial tree, pupillary dilatation

→ Notify ICU. ☎_____
Senior Resident
☎_____

→ **Coma** (See p 128)
→ **Seizures** (See p 142)
→ **Shock** (See p 28)

→ Insert bladder catheter.

Monitor.

(D) **Pralidoxime (2-PAM)**

Adult 1-2 g IV at 0.5 g/min or mixed in 250 ml 0.9 NS over 30 min

Child 25-50 mg/kg diluted to 5% concentration in 0.9 NS over 5-30 min. <u>max.</u> single dose: 2 g May repeat dose after 1 hr and q 6-12 hr if symptoms not relieved. Continuous infusion 10-20 mg/kg/hr

Theophylline Toxicity

Maria Asi-Bautista

> **Consider** theophylline toxicity if
> - Patient received >10 mg/kg theophylline/aminophylline
> - Theophylline level > 20 µg/ml
> - Patients have symptoms of toxicity despite therapeutic levels of theophylline (10-20 µg/ml)
>
> **Suspect** theophylline toxicity in the following patients:
> - Asthmatics on theophylline at home or receiving IV theophylline in the hospital
> - Children with access to theophylline, e.g., accidental ingestions
> - Children with hepatic or cardiac disease treated with theophylline

(A) Severity of **hypokalemia** is proportional to peak serum theophylline levels.

Monitor serial theophylline levels, regardless of an initial low value. This is especially true with slow-release preparations.

(B) **Activated charcoal:** administer sorbitol or magnesium **citrate** only with the first dose. Administer charcoal, even after IV overdose.

GoLYTELY 40 ml/kg/hr PO or per NGT, <u>max</u>. 2 L/hr

(C) Infants are at a greater risk for dysrhythmias.

(D) Seizures can be generalized tonic-clonic, but occasionally are focal and resistant to therapy.

Drugs known to inhibit theophylline metabolism (partial list)	
allopurinol	furosemide
cimetidine	nifedipine
ciprofloxacin	propranolol
erythromycin	verapamil

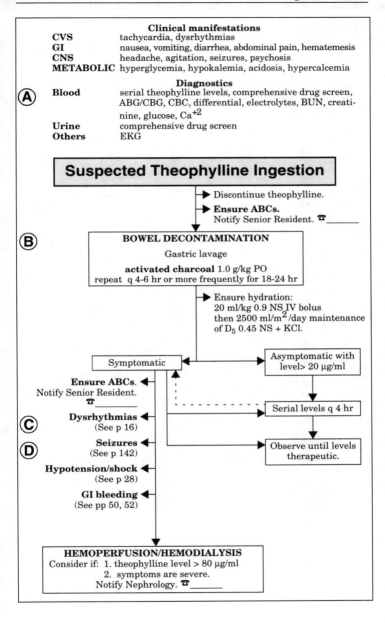

Clinical manifestations

CVS	tachycardia, dysrhythmias
GI	nausea, vomiting, diarrhea, abdominal pain, hematemesis
CNS	headache, agitation, seizures, psychosis
METABOLIC	hyperglycemia, hypokalemia, acidosis, hypercalcemia

Diagnostics

(A)

Blood	serial theophylline levels, comprehensive drug screen, ABG/CBG, CBC, differential, electrolytes, BUN, creatinine, glucose, Ca^{+2}
Urine	comprehensive drug screen
Others	EKG

Suspected Theophylline Ingestion

→ Discontinue theophylline.

→ **Ensure ABCs.**
Notify Senior Resident. ☎_____

(B) **BOWEL DECONTAMINATION**

Gastric lavage

activated charcoal 1.0 g/kg PO
repeat q 4-6 hr or more frequently for 18-24 hr

→ Ensure hydration:
20 ml/kg 0.9 NS IV bolus
then 2500 ml/m^2/day maintenance
of D_5 0.45 NS + KCl.

Symptomatic ← Asymptomatic with level> 20 µg/ml

Ensure ABCs.
Notify Senior Resident.
☎_____

Serial levels q 4 hr

(C) **Dysrhythmias**
(See p 16)

(D) **Seizures**
(See p 142)

Observe until levels therapeutic.

Hypotension/shock
(See p 28)

GI bleeding
(See pp 50, 52)

HEMOPERFUSION/HEMODIALYSIS
Consider if: 1. theophylline level > 80 µg/ml
2. symptoms are severe.
Notify Nephrology. ☎_____

Metabolic

Acute Neonatal Hyperammonemia

Mary Lieh-Lai

> Acute neonatal hyperammonemia generally results from inherited urea cycle enzyme deficiencies. Hyperammonemia is the characteristic biochemical manifestation of these disorders. The clinical signs and symptoms that result are due to the toxic effects of hyperammonemia on the CNS.

(A) Blood for serum ammonia should be obtained as a free-flowing sample. Tourniquet should not be used. Send specimen in heparinized (green top) tube on ice to lab STAT.

(B) Goals of treatment:
1. reducing the circulating levels of urea precursors (including ammonia), as well as the accumulating intermediates
2. reducing the requirement for ureagenesis
3. correcting arginine deficiency when necessary

(C) Disorders of organic acidemias can interfere with the urea cycle enzymes, causing hyperammonemia with high anion gap metabolic acidosis. However, regardless of anion gap, urine organic acids must still be obtained on all patients with hyperammonemia.

(D) Carnitine level: serum should be separated immediately.

(E) **Sodium benzoate** is currently under investigation in the treatment of hyperammonemia. Discuss with Genetics service. ☎_____

The following guidelines are part of the protocol in use at the Children's Hospital of Michigan:
- **sodium benzoate** 250 mg/kg IV loading dose
- **sodium phenylacetate** 250 mg/kg IV loading dose followed by 250 mg/kg/day IV infusion of both until ammonia level returns to near normal.

Oral or IV sodium benzoate rapidly reduces blood ammonia in infants with acute hyperammonemia.

Clinical manifestations

Newborn with vomiting, poor feeding, lethargy, hypothermia, hypotonia (which can be severe) or spasticity, irritability and opisthotonus, tachypnea, grunting respirations

Diagnostics

(A) NH_3, AST, ALT, serum electrolytes, BUN, creatinine, ABG/CBG, Ca^{+2}, anion gap; 7 ml blood in a green-top heparinized tube for plasma amino acid quantitation, and urine for organic acids. Freeze 10-15 ml of urine for further testing. Call appropriate laboratory to process amino acids and urine organic acids ASAP. ☎_____

Suspected Acute Neonatal Hyperammonemia

➤ **Ensure ABCs.**
➤ Notify Genetics. ☎_____

(B) Avoid any form of amino acids or protein intake. Start IV D_{10}0.3 NS + KCl at maintenance rate. Fluid resuscitation: 20 ml/kg 0.9 NS if patient is in hypovolemic shock. (See p 128)

Serum NH_3 > 200 μmol/L

YES ←——————————————→ NO

(B)
Hemodialysis:
Consult Nephrology. ☎_____
Consult Surgery for vascular access. ☎_____
Notify ICU. ☎_____

➤ Continue to monitor. ◄

(B) **Arginine hydrochloride 10% solution**
660 mg/kg IV in 35 ml/kg 10% glucose over 90 min (6 ml/kg) followed by additional 660 mg/kg/24 hr as a continuous infusion

(C) **If anion gap is high**

➤ Obtain serum carnitine level **(D)**
(total and free).

(B) Administer:
• **$NaHCO_3$** 1.0 mEq/kg IV bolus.
  Consider continuous infusion.
• **Biotin** 5 mg PO
• **Carnitine** 100 mg/kg/day PO in 3 doses
  per NG tube
• **Vitamin B_{12}** 1 mg IM q day

Study protocol: discuss with Genetics.
(E) **Sodium benzoate**

Neurologic

Coma

Katherine Ling-McGeorge

> Implies either bilateral hemispheric/cortical dysfunction or brainstem/reticular activating system dysfunction.

Patients with a GCS ≤ 8 should be admitted to the ICU. See p 229.

(A) Seizures have occasionally been observed with the use of **flumazenil**.

(B) Adjunctive therapy: control seizures, correct acid-base abnormalities, thermal regulation, antacids/H₂ blockers, Lacrilube to diminish incidence of corneal dessication.

(C) **Lesion localization and differential diagnosis are imperative to therapy!**

General appearance
level of consciousness

Lethargy	Drowsiness
Obtunded	Blunted
Stupor	Barely arousable
Coma	Unresponsive
Persistent vegetative state	Brainstem function only

Vital signs

↑ Temp	Infection
Tachycardia	Shock, DKA, CHF
Bradycardia ⎫ Hypertension ⎭	Increased ICP, poisoning
Hypotension	Shock, Adrenal failure

Motor exam (cortical function)

> Watch for spontaneous movements. Use **noxious stimuli**: sternal rub or subungual pressure to elicit **posturing**; **repeat** stimuli to validate finding; drop patient's arm on his/her face to elicit voluntary movements.
>
> | | |
> |---|---|
> | Decorticate (arms flexed, abducted) | Cortical dysfunction |
> | Decerebrate (extended extremities) | High brainstem dysfunction |
> | Flaccid / hypotonic | Brainstem dysfunction, any level |
> | Hypertonic | Corticospinal injury |

*(Continued on p 130)

Diagnostics

ABG/CBG, BUN, electrolytes, Ca^{+2}, glucose, comprehensive toxicology screens
Also consider: CBC, differential, coagulation profile, creatinine, osmolality, Mg^{+2}, P, COHb, ammonia, AST, ALT, metabolic screen, EEG, EKG

Comatose Patient

Stabilize C-spine. ◄—► Ensure ABCs.
Protect airway.   Notify Senior Resident. ☎_____

(A) **Immediately correctable**

$D_{25}W$ 1-2 ml/kg IV
naloxone 0.1 mg/kg IV
flumazenil (Romazicon)
 0.2 mg IV over 30 sec
May repeat with 0.3 mg X 1

☆ **Indications for urgent head CT**
Suspected trauma
Bleeding disorders
Focal neurologic signs
Increased ICP
Suspected intracranial mass

Notify Radiology. ☎_____

☆**Increased ICP**
(See p 134)

Hyperventilate.
Head CT with
supervision, when stable

(B) **Adjunctive Therapy**

Signs of Infection☆
(See pp 88, 90)

Lumbar puncture when stable
STAT antibiotics
(may have to precede LP)

History: onset, preceding complaints, trauma, medications and toxins at home
(include medication list of all occupants/visitors to the home)

Skin

Erythema	CO, atropine, mercury
Cyanosis	Hypoxia, CNS emboli in patients with congenial heart disease (R→L shunting)
Petechiae, splinter hemorrhages	Infectious endocarditis, coagulopathy
Icterus, spider angiomata	Hepatic encephalopathy
Periungual fibroma	Tuberous sclerosis
Desquamation	Vitamin A intoxication
Rash	SLE, infection
Pigmentation	Addison's disease
Needle tracks	Drugs

Breath

Fruity	DKA
Garlic	Arsenic, paraldehyde, organophosphates
Almonds	Cyanide
Alcohol	Ethanol

Eyes

Periorbital ecchymosis	Blow-out orbital fracture
Retinal hemorrhages	Shaken baby syndrome
Chemosis	Cavernous sinus thrombosis

Ears

Battle's sign	Basilar skull fracture
Hemotympanum	Trauma
CSF otorrhea	Trauma

Nose

CSF rhinorrhea	Trauma

Mouth

Tongue lacerations	Seizures
Pigmentation	Addison's disease
Gingival lines	Plumbism

Neck

Rigidity	Infection, intracranial bleed
Thyromegaly	Thyrotoxicosis, myxedema

Head

VP shunt	Hydrocephalus, infection

(C) **NEUROLOGIC ASSESSMENT**

Supratentorial	**Subtentorial**	**Psychiatric**	**Metabolic**
Focal cerebral dysfunction	Sudden onset **(D)** Abnormal cold calorics, doll's eyes reflexes	Pupils normal or dilated	Preceding confusion or stupor
Rostrocaudal progression	CN palsies	Unpredictable ocular reflexes	Symmetrical motor signs
Asymmetric motor signs	Abnormal respiratory patterns	Hyperventilation	*Nl pupillary* rxn
Abnormal pupillary reaction **(D)**	**Intubate early!**	No pathologic reflexes Eyelids close actively	Myoclonus, tremor or seizures Acid-base imbalance **(E)**

✳(Continued from 128)

Table 11-1. Brainstem evaluation
- **Pupillary reflex tends to remain intact with metabolic insults. Check drug history!**

Bilateral	Normal/small	Reactive	Toxic/metabolic
	Midposition	Fixed	Midbrain dysfunction (parasympathetic, sympathetic)
	Pinpoint	Reactive	Narcotics, barbiturates, organophosphates
		Fixed	Pontine lesion (sympathetic)
	Large	Reactive	Anticholinergic agents, postictal, metabolic
		Fixed	Toxic/metabolic, anoxic
Unilateral	Small	Minimal	Ipsilateral sympathetic dysfunction
	Large	Fixed	Midbrain or ipsilateral CN III, uncal herniation
Hippus			Midbrain

- **Corneal reflex** CN V sensory, CN VII motor
  Oculocephalic reflex/**Dolls eyes**
  C-spine injury must be ruled out before maneuver.

  Present = eyes appear to gaze forward upon lateral head turning, i.e., eyes deviate to the opposite side of head turning. Reflects absence of cortical influence on the brainstem. Indicates intact brainstem function.

  Oculovestibular reflex/**cold calorics**
  Ascertain integrity of tympanic membranes and ear canals free of cerumen.

  > Elevate head 30°. Place small catheter in the external canal near the tympanic membrane, and introduce ice water slowly from a syringe into the canal of the unresponsive patient. Maximum volume in each ear is about 120 ml. Allow 5 min for the oculovestibular system to stabilize before performing the caloric test in the opposite ear.

  In a normal awake patient: Nystagmus is observed with the slow component toward the irrigated ear, and the fast component away.

  In coma: The fast component disappears, and the eyes tonically deviate toward the irrigated ear. Severe brainstem injury obliterates the response to the cold caloric test.

• Respiratory Patterns

Cheyne-Stokes Bilateral hemispheric dysfunction: transtentorial herniation, DKA, CHF

Hyperventilation Brainstem dysfunction
Metabolic acidosis: DKA, uremia, poisoning, lactic acidosis, salicylates (late)
Respiratory alkalosis: salicylates (early), hepatic encephalopathy
Reye's syndrome

Apneustic Pontine dysfunction

Ataxic/agonal Medullary

Hypoventilation Drugs

(D) Nonmetabolic causes: neoplasia, hemorrhage, CVA, vasculitis

(E) Anoxia/post-CPR, hypoglycemia, DKA, adrenal insufficiency, porphyria, uremia, hepatic encephalopathy, hyperammonemia, Reye's syndrome, inborn errors of metabolism, hyper/hypocalcemia, hyper/hyponatremia, hyper/hypomagnesemia, acidosis/alkalosis, CO_2 narcosis, hyperosmolality, vitamin deficient/dependent states, HUS

Toxins: barbiturates, phenytoin, narcotics, salicylates, lead, cyclic antidepressants, phenothiazines, amphetamines, iron, CO, alcohol, organophosphates, carbamates

Guillain-Barré Syndrome

Mary Lieh-Lai

> An acute, inflammatory peripheral neuropathy, also known as acute
> inflammatory polyradiculoneuropathy. Autoimmune mechanisms are
> implicated as the cause.

(A) Neurologic symptoms are usually preceded by a viral illness, commonly URI or gastroenteritis. Other prodromal diseases: mononucleosis, scarlet fever

(B) Differential diagnoses: heavy metal poisoning, thiamine deficiency, porphyria, botulism, and poliomyelitis

(C) GBS is frequently accompanied by autonomic dysfunction, which results in abnormal peripheral vasomotor tone and cardiac rhythm disturbances. This results in extremes in BP and dysrhythmias, which, however, are usually short-lived, and the temptation to treat these symptoms should be tempered by the fact that pharmacologic agents can worsen the autonomic dysfunction.

(D) The administration of depolarizing agents to patients with GBS is associated with **ventricular dysrhythmias**. Use of sedative and anesthetic agents can accentuate autonomic instability.

(E) Because of muscle weakness, these patients are prone to decubitus ulcers, deep vein thrombosis, and pulmonary embolism. In addition, urinary retention often leads to UTIs. A decreased respiratory effort leads to pneumonia in 2/3 of patients with GBS. Continued management should take these into account, and supportive therapy should be directed toward the prevention of these complications.

(A) **Motor:**
Clinical manifestations
Symmetric weakness in the lower extremities, typically distal musculature, followed by progressive ascending paralysis

Sensory: Symptoms (numbness or paresthesias) usually occur early. Patients typically present with inability to walk or generalized weakness.

Other symptoms: Cranial nerve palsies, cerebellar ataxia. 10% of patients present with upper extremity weakness. A third present without any sensory deficits.

Physical findings
Areflexia, muscle weakness, CN palsies, altered level of consciousness, urinary retention, loss of vibratory and/or position sense. Weakness progresses over 2-14 days. A third develop respiratory muscle weakness leading to respiratory failure.

NOTE: **Patients with GBS in respiratory failure will not show signs and symptoms of respiratory distress (retractions, etc.) because of muscle weakness.**

Diagnostics
"Albuminocytologic dissociation":
CSF protein is elevated in the absence of pleocytosis.

EMG: delayed nerve conduction
FVC: every 2-4 hr to monitor for onset of respiratory failure.
ABG/CBG, pulse oximeter
Frequent neuro
checks: level of consciousness, gag and cough reflex, ability to swallow
Hemodynamic
status: monitor HR, heart rhythm, BP, and temperature.

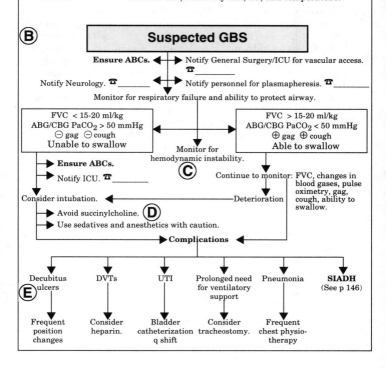

(B)

Suspected GBS

Ensure ABCs. ◄——► Notify General Surgery/ICU for vascular access. ☎ ____

Notify Neurology. ☎ ____ ◄——► Notify personnel for plasmapheresis. ☎ ____

Monitor for respiratory failure and ability to protect airway.

| FVC < 15-20 ml/kg
ABG/CBG $PaCO_2$ > 50 mmHg
⊖ gag ⊖ cough
Unable to swallow | | FVC > 15-20 ml/kg
ABG/CBG $PaCO_2$ < 50 mmHg
⊕ gag ⊕ cough
Able to swallow |

Ensure ABCs.
Notify ICU. ☎ ____

Monitor for hemodynamic instability. **(C)**

Continue to monitor: FVC, changes in blood gases, pulse oximetry, gag, cough, ability to swallow.

Consider intubation. ◄———————— Deterioration

Avoid succinylcholine. **(D)**
Use sedatives and anesthetics with caution.

——► **Complications** ◄——

(E) Decubitus ulcers | DVTs | UTI | Prolonged need for ventilatory support | Pneumonia | **SIADH** (See p 146)

Frequent position changes | Consider heparin. | Bladder catheterization q shift | Consider tracheostomy. | Frequent chest physiotherapy

Increased Intracranial Pressure

Alexandre Rotta

> Increased ICP can result in brain herniation. The increased ICP and brainstem compression results in a progressive deterioration in the level of consciousness, and if untreated, may lead to apnea and death.

(A) **History:** bleeding disorders, behavioral changes, CNS infection, hypertension, vision changes, stroke, trauma, chemotherapy, diabetic patient undergoing fluid resuscitation for DKA, mismanagement of other hyperosmolar states

Physical exam: look for retinal hemorrhages, meningeal signs, depressed skull fracture.

(B) Ventilate at 10-20 breaths/min above normal respiratory rate for age. Aim for $PaCO_2$ 25-30 mmHg. A lower $PaCO_2$ may, however, be necessary for short periods of time during acute ICP elevation.

(C) Under sterile conditions, puncture reservoir with 25-gauge butterfly needle, and check column of CSF to assess pressure. Slowly aspirate aliquots of 5-10 ml CSF. Send CSF for labs. **Senior Resident or Neurosurgeon must be present.**

For ventricular tap, consult Neurosurgery. ☎ _____

(D) **Vasogenic edema:** disrupted blood-brain barrier with increased cerebral vascular permeability seen with tumors, trauma, hemorrhage, inflammation (meningitis, abscess)

Cytotoxic edema: cell death or failure of the Na-ATPase pump, generating fluid shift to the intracellular space, seen with water intoxication, hypoxic-ischemic injury

Interstitial edema: increase in CSF hydrostatic pressure with CSF shift to the interstitial space seen with obstructive hydrocephalus or shunt malfunction

Mass: neoplastic, cystic, vascular, abscess

(E) **Pentobarbital:** 2 mg/kg IV q 2-3 hr

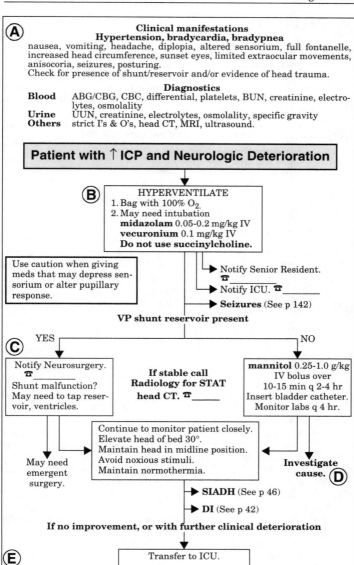

(A)
Clinical manifestations
Hypertension, bradycardia, bradypnea
nausea, vomiting, headache, diplopia, altered sensorium, full fontanelle, increased head circumference, sunset eyes, limited extraocular movements, anisocoria, seizures, posturing.
Check for presence of shunt/reservoir and/or evidence of head trauma.

Diagnostics
Blood ABG/CBG, CBC, differential, platelets, BUN, creatinine, electrolytes, osmolality
Urine UUN, creatinine, electrolytes, osmolality, specific gravity
Others strict I's & O's, head CT, MRI, ultrasound.

Patient with ↑ ICP and Neurologic Deterioration

(B) HYPERVENTILATE
1. Bag with 100% O_2.
2. May need intubation
midazolam 0.05-0.2 mg/kg IV
vecuronium 0.1 mg/kg IV
Do not use succinylcholine.

Use caution when giving meds that may depress sensorium or alter pupillary response.

→ Notify Senior Resident. ☎_____
→ Notify ICU. ☎_____
→ **Seizures** (See p 142)

VP shunt reservoir present

(C) YES   NO

Notify Neurosurgery. ☎___
Shunt malfunction?
May need to tap reservoir, ventricles.

If stable call
Radiology for STAT
head CT. ☎_____

mannitol 0.25-1.0 g/kg
IV bolus over
10-15 min q 2-4 hr
Insert bladder catheter.
Monitor labs q 4 hr.

May need emergent surgery.

Continue to monitor patient closely.
Elevate head of bed 30°.
Maintain head in midline position.
Avoid noxious stimuli.
Maintain normothermia.

Investigate cause. (D)

→ **SIADH** (See p 46)
→ **DI** (See p 42)

If no improvement, or with further clinical deterioration

(E) Transfer to ICU.
Continue neuroresuscitation

Myasthenia Gravis

Alexandre Rotta

> Disorder of neuromuscular transmission (including voluntary muscle), due to a decrease in number or function of acetylcholine receptors.

(A) May be atypical and hard to differentiate. Edrophonium test may be necessary.

(B)

Drugs to avoid in patients with MG	
Analgesics	meperidine, morphine
Anesthetics	lidocaine, procaine
Antiarrhythmics	procainamide, quinidine, quinine (including tonic water)
Antibiotics	gentamicin, kanamycin, polymixins, streptomycin, tetracycline, tobramycin
Anticonvulsants	carbamazepine, phenytoin, valproic acid
Anxiolytics	benzodiazepines
Muscle relaxants	baclofen
Paralyzing agents	curare, succinylcholine

(C) FVC, ABG/CBG, pulse oximeter, CR monitor. See p 228 for normal values. Follow ABG/CBG if unable to obtain FVC. Pulse oximetry may not be reliable as a monitoring device, because hypoxemia occurs much later.

(D) Differential diagnoses of MG:
> infections and their sequelae or related conditions: polio, coxsackie, echovirus, GBS, transverse myelitis, acute cerebellar ataxia, acute infectious myositis, diphtheric neuropathy, rabies
> neuromuscular blockade: botulism, tick paralysis, drugs
> periodic paralysis: hyper/hypo and normokalemic periodic paralysis, acute intermittent porphyria
> intoxication: heavy metals, INH, steroids, vincristine, nitrofurantoin
> spinal cord: mass, trauma, vascular malformation, vasculitis, occult dysraphic states

(E) Maternal and newborn samples (in transient neonatal MG). Antibody absent in persistent neonatal MG. Results not available immediately.

(F) Mother must have MG; transplacental maternal anti-ACh receptor antibody is implicated. Symptoms occur early: hours, days after birth.

(G) Similar to adult MG, age of onset usually > 8 yr, waxes and wanes, may be associated with seizures

(H) Mother is disease-free. Patient with diffuse weakness with pronounced cranial nerve involvement. Can be autosomal recessive, often mild; remission is rare. Absent anti-ACh receptor antibodies. Often resistant to therapy.

(I) **Pyridostigmine:** IV dose is 1/30th of PO dose. Onset 10-40 min, duration 3-12 hr.
Neostigmine: IV dose is 1/15th of PO dose. Onset 10-20 min, duration 3-4 hr.

(J) ☎ _____ Consult Surgery or ICU for large caliber IV access.

Consult personnel responsible for plasmapheresis.

(K) **Prednisone** 20-30 mg/m^2 PO q other day. May need to increase dose.

(A)

	Clinical setting	Clinical manifestations	Treatment
Myasthenic crisis	infection, menses, surgery, stress *under*medication, tolerance, hazardous meds (B)	muscle weakness, mydriasis, tachycardia, absence of fasciculations ☆**Improvement** with edrophonium	AChe therapy may need ventilatory support.
Cholinergic crisis	*over*medication with AChe	diarrhea, cramps, diaphoresis, muscle weakness, miosis, bradycardia, fasciculations, salivation ☆**Worsening** with edrophonium	**withhold** AChe consider atropine. may need ventilatory support.

Patient with Suspected MG

(C)

(D)

Close monitoring of respiratory status: pulse oximeter CR monitor check FVC, ABG/CBG

Acute respiratory failure (See p 170)

← → Consider differential diagnosis.

► **Ensure ABCs.** Signs/symptoms of respiratory distress may not manifest, because of weakness.

(E) —————— Diagnostics ——————

Labs ACh receptor antibody	☆**edrophonium (Tensilon)** test (Notify Neurology before performing.) Monitor BP and HR. Double blind fashion. Use 0.9 NS as placebo **Tensilon** 0.15 mg/kg/dose IV/IM/SC (<u>max</u>. 10 mg) over 3 min. Assess for increased strength and FVC in approx. 1 min. Drug effect lasts approx. 6 min. Have **atropine** available 0.02 mg/kg/dose IV (<u>min</u>. 0.1 mg, max. 2.0 mg) for severe bradycardia, hypotension, cramps.	**Studies** EMG

Classification and Management of MG

(F)

Neonatal MG ———

► Anticholinesterase therapy: **pyridostigmine** (Mestinon) 7 mg/kg/day PO ÷ q 4-6 hr **neostigmine** (Prostigmin) 2 mg/kg/day PO ÷ q 4-6 hr

(G)

Juvenile MG ———

{ Double volume exchange transfusion (See p 203) Plasmapheresis (J) }

► Thymectomy

(H)

Neonatal persistent MG (Congenital) ———

► Steroids (K), consider IV gamma globulin.

► AChe therapy (I)

► **ephedrine** 0.4-0.8 mg/kg/dose PO q 4-6 hr Onset 15-40 min, duration 4-6 hr

Spinal Cord Injury

Mary Lieh-Lai

(A) Epidemiology: traumatic SCI accounts for about 12,000 paraplegic and quadriplegic patients in the US. Major causes include motor vehicle accidents (50%), falls, and sports injuries (including diving). There is a higher incidence in males 15-35 years of age. SCI should be suspected and assumed to be present in any child who has sustained multiple traumatic injury.

Upon stabilization of a patient who is suspected to have SCI, a complete detailed neurologic examination must be carried out to help determine the level and extent of injury. Include assessment and documentation of motor, sensory, and reflex function (including perianal sensation and voluntary rectal sphincter control). (See p 140 for dermatomes.)

(B) The goals of radiographic examination of a patient with suspected SCI are:

1. To detect and characterize the type and extent of bony fractures, subluxation, or dislocation.
2. If the patient has neurologic deficits, radiographs may help differentiate intrinsic and extrinsic spinal lesions that may require surgical decompression.

Plain films (See p 141 for algorithm on imaging)

1. Cross-table lateral view of the neck taken with patient immobilized and still on the trauma board. The radiograph should show the C7-T1 articulation.
2. Additional plain films (obtained after patient stabilization): AP view of the neck, odontoid or open mouth view, and bilateral oblique positions.
3. Consider plain films of the thoracolumbosacral spine in all patients with severe trauma, those who are unconscious, and/or if injury to the lower spinal cord is suspected.

(C) Spinal cord stabilization: should allow for restoration of the patient to an immobilized neutral supine position, as well as allow personnel access to the patient for maintenance of airway and circulation.

1. Place patient on straight backboard: maintain alignment of the head and neck to the axis of the body.
2. Apply cervical collar and towel rolls or sandbags, one on each side of the head.
3. By applying tape or Velcro straps to the forehead, chest (do not restrict breathing), pelvis, knees, and ankles, complete patient immobilization is achieved.
4. Special consideration: infants have disproportionately larger heads, such that when they are placed on flat backboards, anterior flexion of the head and neck occurs. Effective ways to prevent this include modification of the backboard to provide a recess for the occiput, or double mattress pads to raise the trunk.

*(Continued on p 140)

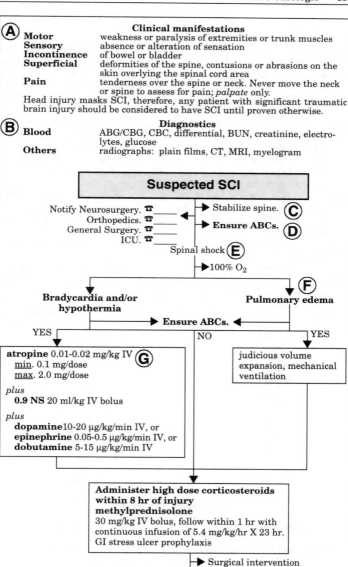

(A) **Clinical manifestations**

Motor	weakness or paralysis of extremities or trunk muscles
Sensory	absence or alteration of sensation
Incontinence	of bowel or bladder
Superficial	deformities of the spine, contusions or abrasions on the skin overlying the spinal cord area
Pain	tenderness over the spine or neck. Never move the neck or spine to assess for pain; *palpate* only.

Head injury masks SCI, therefore, any patient with significant traumatic brain injury should be considered to have SCI until proven otherwise.

(B) **Diagnostics**

Blood	ABG/CBG, CBC, differential, BUN, creatinine, electrolytes, glucose
Others	radiographs: plain films, CT, MRI, myelogram

Suspected SCI

Notify Neurosurgery. ☎ _____
Orthopedics. ☎ _____
General Surgery. ☎ _____
ICU. ☎ _____

→ Stabilize spine. **(C)**
→ Ensure ABCs. **(D)**

Spinal shock **(E)**

→ 100% O_2

(F)

Bradycardia and/or hypothermia —— **Pulmonary edema**

→ **Ensure ABCs.** ←

YES | NO | YES

atropine 0.01-0.02 mg/kg IV **(G)**
<u>min</u>. 0.1 mg/dose
<u>max</u>. 2.0 mg/dose

plus
0.9 NS 20 ml/kg IV bolus

plus
dopamine 10-20 µg/kg/min IV, or
epinephrine 0.05-0.5 µg/kg/min IV, or
dobutamine 5-15 µg/kg/min IV

judicious volume expansion, mechanical ventilation

Administer high dose corticosteroids within 8 hr of injury
methylprednisolone
30 mg/kg IV bolus, follow within 1 hr with continuous infusion of 5.4 mg/kg/hr X 23 hr.
GI stress ulcer prophylaxis

→ Surgical intervention if necessary

(H) Supportive care and rehabilitation

✻(Continued from p 138)

(D) Intubation of a patient with suspected SCI should be performed with the child in a neutral position. Manual in-line axial traction may sometimes be necessary. If the patient does not require immediate intubation, frequent monitoring (ABG/CBG) is essential to detect respiratory failure and institute appropriate intervention.

(E) With SCI, the sympathetic outflow tracts may be disrupted. This results in a loss of vasomotor tone, peripheral vasodilation, pooling of blood in the capacitance vessels, and hypotension. Additionally, disruption of sympathetic tracts leads to bradycardia and other dysrhythmias, which further reduce cardiac output.

(F) SCI is associated with pulmonary edema, the mechanism of which is unclear, but may result from a massive sympathetic discharge, which leads to a disruption of pulmonary capillary endothelium.

(G) If bradycardia persists despite atropine, the patient may need a cardiac pacemaker.

(H) Supportive care: respiratory support, GI stress ulcer prophylaxis, nutritional support, prevention of decubitus ulcers, bowel and bladder care, physical therapy and rehabilitation

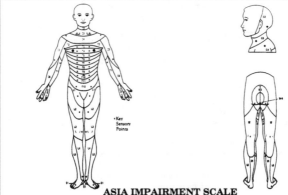

ASIA IMPAIRMENT SCALE
(modified from Frankel)

A = Complete. No sensory or motor function is preserved in the scral segments S4-S5

B = Incomplete. Sensory but not motor function is preserved below the neurological level and extends through the scral segments S4-S5.

C = Incomplete. Motor function is preserved below the neurological level, and the majority of key muscles below the neurological level, have muscle grade less than 3.

D = Incomplete. Motor function is preserved below the neurological level, and the majority of key muscles below the neurological level have a muscle grade greater than or equal to 3.

E = Normal. Sensory and motor function is normal.

From American Spinal Injury Association. *Standards for Neurological Classification of Spinal Injury Patients,* **Atlanta: American Spinal Injury Association, 1990, p 199. With permission.**

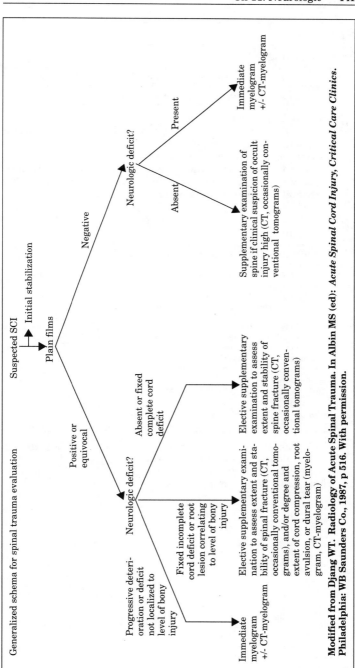

Generalized schema for spinal trauma evaluation

Suspected SCI

Initial stabilization

Plain films

Positive or equivocal

Neurologic deficit?

- Progressive deterioration or deficit not localized to level of bony injury

  Immediate myelogram +/- CT-myelogram

- Fixed incomplete cord deficit or root lesion correlating to level of bony injury

  Elective supplementary examination to assess extent and stability of spinal fracture (CT, occasionally conventional tomograms), and/or degree and extent of cord compression, root avulsion, or dural tear (myelogram, CT-myelogram)

- Absent or fixed complete cord deficit

  Elective supplementary examination to assess extent and stability of spine fracture (CT, occasionally conventional tomograms)

Negative

Neurologic deficit?

- Present

  Immediate myelogram +/- CT-myelogram

- Absent

  Supplementary examination of spine if clinical suspicion of occult injury high (CT, occasionally conventional tomograms)

Modified from Djang WT. Radiology of Acute Spinal Trauma. In Albin MS (ed): *Acute Spinal Cord Injury, Critical Care Clinics.* Philadelphia: WB Saunders Co, 1987, p 516. With permission.

Status Epilepticus

Frederick Klingbeil

> Status epilepticus is a neurologic disorder characterized by continuous generalized or focal seizures lasting > 15 min or a series of seizures lasting > 30 min without the patient regaining consciousness.

(A) Indications for CT scan
head trauma, evidence of increased ICP, focal neurologic deficit, focal seizure activity

Contraindications for spinal tap
known or suspected increased ICP, focal neurologic deficit, cardiopulmonary instability, severe coagulopathy, thrombocytopenia, infection over tap site

(B)

Causes of status epilepticus
Idiopathic
Fever, e.g., complex febrile seizure
Anticonvulsant medication withdrawal, poor compliance with medications
Head trauma, CVA, encephalopathy, tumor, intracranial hemorrhage, shunt malfunction
HUS, other causes of acute renal failure
Hypoxia, hyponatremia, hypernatremia, hypoglycemia, hypomagnesemia, hypocalcemia, hepatic failure, inherited disorders
Alcohol, theophylline, cyclosporine, lead intoxication, other drug ingestions
Meningitis, encephalitis

Life-threatening complications		
aspiration	airway obstruction	respiratory acidosis
apnea	hypoxemia	pulmonary edema
		increased cerebral metabolic rate

(C) If IV access is not available, use **rectal paraldehyde** 0.3 ml/kg in equal amount of mineral oil. <u>max</u>. 5 ml

May consider **diazepam** 0.3 mg/kg PR or per endotracheal tube. <u>max</u>. 5 mg.

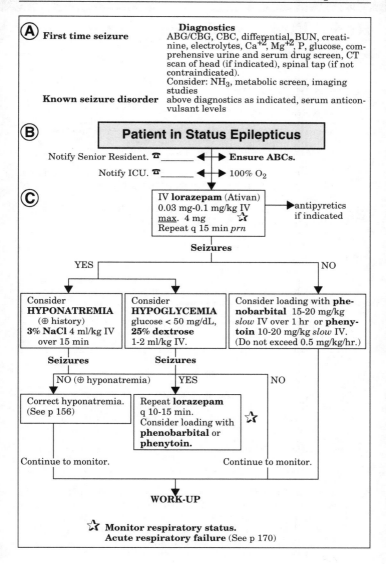

(A) **First time seizure**

Diagnostics
ABG/CBG, CBC, differential, BUN, creatinine, electrolytes, Ca^{+2}, Mg^{+2}, P, glucose, comprehensive urine and serum drug screen, CT scan of head (if indicated), spinal tap (if not contraindicated).
Consider: NH_3, metabolic screen, imaging studies

Known seizure disorder above diagnostics as indicated, serum anticonvulsant levels

(B)

Patient in Status Epilepticus

Notify Senior Resident. ☎_____ ◄──► **Ensure ABCs.**

Notify ICU. ☎_____ ◄──► 100% O_2

(C)

IV **lorazepam** (Ativan)
0.03 mg-0.1 mg/kg IV
<u>max</u>. 4 mg   ☆
Repeat q 15 min *prn*
──► antipyretics if indicated

Seizures

YES ──────────────────────── NO

Consider
HYPONATREMIA
(⊕ history)
3% NaCl 4 ml/kg IV
over 15 min

Consider
HYPOGLYCEMIA
glucose < 50 mg/dL,
25% dextrose
1-2 ml/kg IV.

Consider loading with **phenobarbital** 15-20 mg/kg *slow* IV over 1 hr or **phenytoin** 10-20 mg/kg *slow* IV. (Do not exceed 0.5 mg/kg/hr.)

Seizures   **Seizures**

NO (⊕ hyponatremia)   YES   NO

Correct hyponatremia.
(See p 156)

Repeat **lorazepam**
q 10-15 min.
Consider loading with
phenobarbital or
phenytoin.   ☆

Continue to monitor.   Continue to monitor.

WORK-UP

☆ **Monitor respiratory status.**
Acute respiratory failure (See p 170)

Renal Fluids and Electrolytes

Acute Renal Failure

Michelle Rotta

> Acute renal failure is the sudden cessation of bilateral kidney function leading to the accumulation of nitrogenous waste substances, and electrolyte and acid-base imbalance with or without oliguria.

(A) Signs and symptoms usually provide clues to diagnosis. Look for transplantation scars, note pain over scar, signs of infection, and abdominal mass.

(B) May observe abnormal levels of BUN, K, creatinine, Ca^{+2}, P, Mg^{+2}, uric acid, Hb, pH, CO_2 content.

(C)

Pediatric population at risk for acute renal failure
1. Postcardiac surgery (especially in the neonatal period)
2. Postcardiac arrest/shock
3. Sepsis alone and associated with other diseases, e.g., sickle cell disease, bone marrow transplant, malignancies
4. Patients who have undergone renal transplantation
5. Patients with malignancies and tumor lysis syndrome
6. Others: HUS, autoimmune diseases (SLE, JRA), postinfectious glomerulonephritis
7. Hypovolemia

(D)

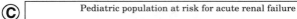

Exogenous nephrotoxic agents (partial list)			
acetaminophen	carbamazepine	Mg^{+2}	P
acyclovir	CO	methanol	prednisone
aminoglycosides	cocaine	NSAIDs (ibuprofen)	rifampin
amoxicillin	ethylene glycol	opioids	sulfonamides
amphotericin B	furosemide	penicillin	tetracyclines
ascorbic acid	heavy metals	phosphates	x-ray contrast media

(E) Replace fluid losses/restore fluid volume **despite** anuric phase. If the only cause of anuria or oliguria is fluid depletion, fluid resuscitation should restore urine flow within six hours or less. Look for ongoing losses if acute renal failure persists in spite of volume expansion.

Consider CVP monitoring to assess fluid status.

(F)

Causes of post-renal oliguria: obstruction	
Urethral:	posterior urethral valves, phimosis, stricture
Bladder:	neurogenic, clots, malignancies, calculi
Ureteral:	*intrinsic*: clot, calculi, stenosis, hydronephrosis
	extrinsic: malignancy, ligation, radiation therapy

✳(Continued on p 146)

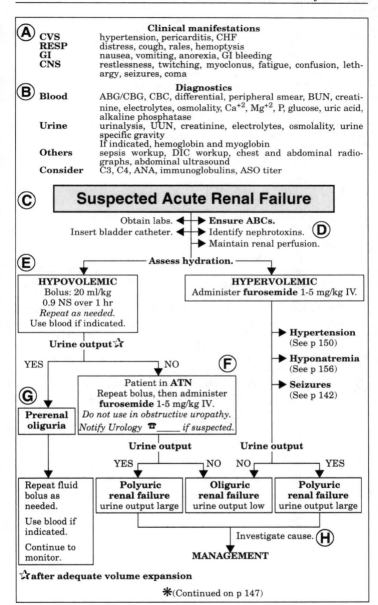

(A) **Clinical manifestations**

CVS	hypertension, pericarditis, CHF
RESP	distress, cough, rales, hemoptysis
GI	nausea, vomiting, anorexia, GI bleeding
CNS	restlessness, twitching, myoclonus, fatigue, confusion, lethargy, seizures, coma

(B) **Diagnostics**

Blood	ABG/CBG, CBC, differential, peripheral smear, BUN, creatinine, electrolytes, osmolality, Ca^{+2}, Mg^{+2}, P, glucose, uric acid, alkaline phosphatase
Urine	urinalysis, UUN, creatinine, electrolytes, osmolality, urine specific gravity If indicated, hemoglobin and myoglobin
Others	sepsis workup, DIC workup, chest and abdominal radiographs, abdominal ultrasound
Consider	C3, C4, ANA, immunoglobulins, ASO titer

(C) ## Suspected Acute Renal Failure

Obtain labs. ◄──► **Ensure ABCs.**
Insert bladder catheter. ◄──► Identify nephrotoxins. **(D)**
──► Maintain renal perfusion.

(E) ──── **Assess hydration.** ────

HYPOVOLEMIC
Bolus: 20 ml/kg
0.9 NS over 1 hr
Repeat as needed.
Use blood if indicated.

HYPERVOLEMIC
Administer **furosemide** 1-5 mg/kg IV.

──► **Hypertension**
(See p 150)

──► **Hyponatremia**
(See p 156)

──► **Seizures**
(See p 142)

Urine output ☆

YES ── ──NO   **(F)**

(G)

Patient in **ATN**
Repeat bolus, then administer
furosemide 1-5 mg/kg IV.
Do not use in obstructive uropathy.
Notify Urology ☎ ____ *if suspected.*

Prerenal
oliguria

Urine output   **Urine output**
YES ── ──NO   NO── ──YES

Repeat fluid bolus as needed. Use blood if indicated. Continue to monitor.	**Polyuric renal failure** urine output large	**Oliguric renal failure** urine output low	**Polyuric renal failure** urine output large

Investigate cause. **(H)**

MANAGEMENT

☆**after adequate volume expansion**

✱(Continued on p 147)

✳(Continued from 144)

G

> Causes of pre-renal oliguria leading to renal hypoperfusion
>
> - true hypovolemia: dehydration, hemorrhage, third spacing, e.g., postoperative, burns
> - relative hypovolemia: septic shock, anaphylaxis
> - decreased cardiac output: CHF, myocarditis
> - renal ischemia: surgery, trauma, renal artery thrombosis, e.g., UAC placement

H

> Causes of acute renal failure due to renal disease
> - nephrotoxin (tubular damage)
>   A. *Endogenous*: myoglobin, hemoglobin, uric acid, calcium, phosphorus, oxalate, xanthine
>
>   B. *Exogenous*: see Table **D**
> - vasculitic diseases: PAN, SLE, HUS, DIC, TTP
> - immunologic diseases (glomerular damage)
>   SLE, glomerulonephritis, nephrotic syndrome, Goodpasture's syndrome
> - interstitial: infectious, infiltrative, malignancy, sarcoidosis

MYOGLOBINURIA may be seen secondary to rhabdomyolysis or crush injuries. Urinalysis is usually *positive* by reagent strips for blood (myoglobin), but *negative* for RBC microscopically. Administer **mannitol** 0.25 g/kg IV q 6 hr; alkalinize urine with **NaHCO$_3$** IV or ensure adequate hydration and urine output (approximately > 2 ml/kg/hr)

I The goal of therapy is to maintain a stable serum Na$^+$ and a decrease in total body weight by 0.5-1% per day.

J Consider oral phosphate binders or Ca^{+2} supplements.
CaCO$_3$ 25 mEq elemental calcium/kg PO q 6 hr.

K Administer: **NaHCO$_3$** 1 mEq/kg IV over 1 hr,
correct remaining deficit over
8-24 hr. **NaHCO$_3$** tablets
(650 mg = 8 mEq HCO$_3^-$)

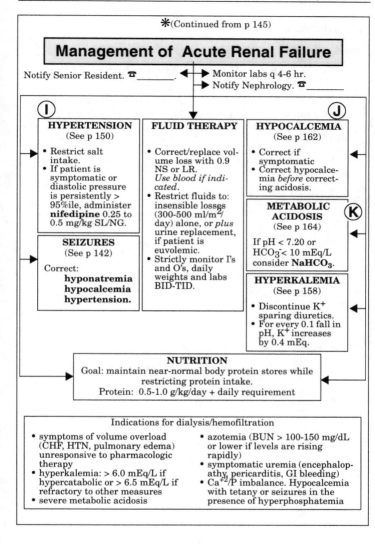

✱(Continued from p 145)

Management of Acute Renal Failure

Notify Senior Resident. ☎_____. ◀━━▶ Monitor labs q 4-6 hr.
━▶ Notify Nephrology. ☎_____

Ⓘ   Ⓙ

HYPERTENSION
(See p 150)

• Restrict salt intake.
• If patient is symptomatic or diastolic pressure is persistently > 95%ile, administer **nifedipine** 0.25 to 0.5 mg/kg SL/NG.

FLUID THERAPY

• Correct/replace volume loss with 0.9 NS or LR. *Use blood if indicated.*
• Restrict fluids to: insensible losses (300-500 ml/m^2/day) alone, or *plus* urine replacement, if patient is euvolemic.
• Strictly monitor I's and O's, daily weights and labs BID-TID.

HYPOCALCEMIA
(See p 162)

• Correct if symptomatic
• Correct hypocalcemia *before* correcting acidosis.

METABOLIC ACIDOSIS Ⓚ
(See p 164)

If pH < 7.20 or HCO_3^-< 10 mEq/L consider **NaHCO₃**.

SEIZURES
(See p 142)

Correct:

**hyponatremia
hypocalcemia
hypertension.**

HYPERKALEMIA
(See p 158)

• Discontinue K^+ sparing diuretics.
• For every 0.1 fall in pH, K^+ increases by 0.4 mEq.

NUTRITION
Goal: maintain near-normal body protein stores while restricting protein intake.
Protein: 0.5-1.0 g/kg/day + daily requirement

Indications for dialysis/hemofiltration

• symptoms of volume overload (CHF, HTN, pulmonary edema) unresponsive to pharmacologic therapy
• hyperkalemia: > 6.0 mEq/L if hypercatabolic or > 6.5 mEq/L if refractory to other measures
• severe metabolic acidosis

• azotemia (BUN > 100-150 mg/dL or lower if levels are rising rapidly)
• symptomatic uremia (encephalopathy, pericarditis, GI bleeding)
• Ca^{+2}/P imbalance. Hypocalcemia with tetany or seizures in the presence of hyperphosphatemia

Hemolytic Uremic Syndrome

Michelle Rotta

> HUS is a disease triad consisting of acute microangiopathic hemolytic anemia, thrombocytopenia, and renal failure

(A) HUS is commonly seen in previously healthy infants and young children who present with signs of acute renal failure, fluid overload, dehydration, hypertension, encephalopathy, anemia. The history often reveals a prodrome of bloody diarrhea, URI, nausea, or vomiting.

Inquire about history of familial or recurrent HUS and of hemolytic anemia.

(B) Typical laboratory findings:

hemoglobin	5-9 g/dl	smear	red cell fragments
platelets	20,000-100,000/mm^3	reticulocytes	moderately increased
Coomb's test	negative	LDH	increased
PT, PTT	usually normal	urinalysis	low-grade hematuria
electrolytes	hyponatremia	stool culture	verotoxin may be ⊕
	hyperkalemia		
	azotemia		
	metabolic acidosis		

Likely organisms: *Escherichia coli* 0157.H7, viral, *Shigella, Salmonella*

(C)

Differential diagnosis
- meningococcemia
- TTP—primarily seen in adults. Neurologic symptoms are more pronounced. Renal involvement is less. No diarrheal prodrome
- disseminated intravascular coagulation—abnormal PT, PTT, fibrinogen Associated primary condition
- nonimmune hemolytic anemia
- bilateral renal vein thrombosis

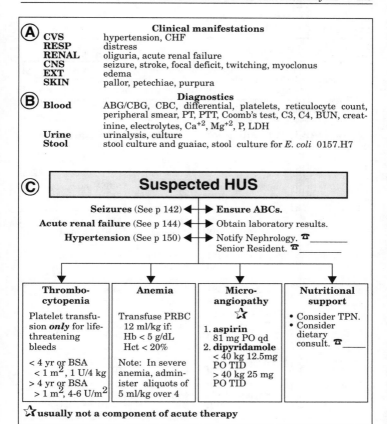

(A)

	Clinical manifestations
CVS	hypertension, CHF
RESP	distress
RENAL	oliguria, acute renal failure
CNS	seizure, stroke, focal deficit, twitching, myoclonus
EXT	edema
SKIN	pallor, petechiae, purpura

(B)

	Diagnostics
Blood	ABG/CBG, CBC, differential, platelets, reticulocyte count, peripheral smear, PT, PTT, Coomb's test, C3, C4, BUN, creatinine, electrolytes, Ca^{+2}, Mg^{+2}, P, LDH
Urine	urinalysis, culture
Stool	stool culture and guaiac, stool culture for *E. coli* 0157.H7

(C)

Suspected HUS

Seizures (See p 142) ◄─► Ensure ABCs.

Acute renal failure (See p 144) ◄─► Obtain laboratory results.

Hypertension (See p 150) ◄─► Notify Nephrology. ☎_____
Senior Resident. ☎_____

Thrombo-cytopenia	**Anemia**	**Micro-angiopathy** ☆	**Nutritional support**
Platelet transfusion *only* for life-threatening bleeds	Transfuse PRBC 12 ml/kg if: Hb < 5 g/dL Hct < 20%	1. **aspirin** 81 mg PO qd	• Consider TPN. • Consider dietary consult. ☎____
< 4 yr or BSA < 1 m², 1 U/4 kg > 4 yr or BSA > 1 m², 4-6 U/m²	Note: In severe anemia, administer aliquots of 5 ml/kg over 4	2. **dipyridamole** < 40 kg 12.5mg PO TID > 40 kg 25 mg PO TID	

☆ usually not a component of acute therapy

Hypertensive Crisis

Katherine Ling-McGeorge

> Hypertensive encephalopathy represents a breakdown in cerebral autoregulation; arterioles are unable to maintain constant cerebral blood flow in response to fluctuations in mean systemic arterial pressure. The hypertensive crisis is usually accompanied by characteristic signs and symptoms.

(A) **Table 12-1. Classification of hypertension by age group**

	Age	Significant	Severe
Newborn	7 days 8-30 days	SBP ≥ 96 mmHg SBP ≥ 104 mmHg	SBP ≥ 106 mmHg SBP ≥ 110 mmHg
Infant	< 2 years	SBP ≥ 112 mmHg DBP ≥ 74 mmHg	SBP ≥ 118 mmHg DBP ≥ 82 mmHg
Children	3-5 years	SBP ≥ 116 mmHg DBP ≥ 76 mmHg	SBP ≥ 124 mmHg DBP ≥ 84 mmHg
	6-9 years	SBP ≥ 122 mmHg DBP ≥ 78 mmHg	SBP ≥ 130 mmHg DBP ≥ 86 mmHg
	10-12 years	SBP ≥ 126 mmHg DBP ≥ 82 mmHg	SBP ≥ 134 mmHg DBP ≥ 90 mmHg
Adolescent	13-15 years	SBP ≥ 136 mmHg DBP ≥ 86 mmHg	SBP ≥ 144 mmHg DBP ≥ 92 mmHg
	16-18 years	SBP ≥ 142 mmHg DBP ≥ 92 mmHg	SBP ≥ 150 mmHg DBP ≥ 98 mmHg

From National Heart, Lung and Blood Institute. *The Report of the Second Task Force on Blood Pressure in Children.* Reproduced by permission of *Pediatrics,* 79:7, 1987.

(B) Additional labs: renin level, aldosterone, ESR, ANA, complement, ASO titer, thyroid studies, cholesterol/triglycerides, uric acid
Additional imaging: abdominal US, echocardiogram, ^{99}Tc-DMSA scan, VCUG

(C) The width of the inner bladder of the BP cuff should approximate 2/3 of the length of the patient's humerus.

✳(Continued on p 152)

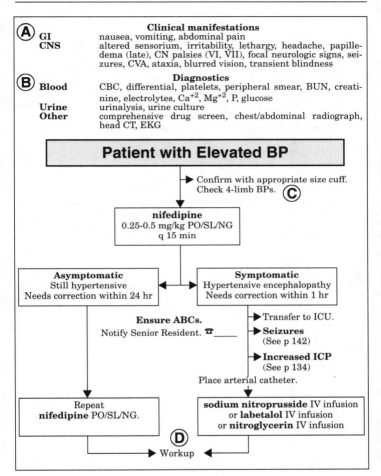

(A) GI
CNS

Clinical manifestations

nausea, vomiting, abdominal pain

altered sensorium, irritability, lethargy, headache, papilledema (late), CN palsies (VI, VII), focal neurologic signs, seizures, CVA, ataxia, blurred vision, transient blindness

(B) Blood

Urine
Other

Diagnostics

CBC, differential, platelets, peripheral smear, BUN, creatinine, electrolytes, Ca^{+2}, Mg^{+2}, P, glucose

urinalysis, urine culture

comprehensive drug screen, chest/abdominal radiograph, head CT, EKG

Patient with Elevated BP

→ Confirm with appropriate size cuff.
Check 4-limb BPs. **(C)**

nifedipine
0.25-0.5 mg/kg PO/SL/NG
q 15 min

| **Asymptomatic**
Still hypertensive
Needs correction within 24 hr | **Symptomatic**
Hypertensive encephalopathy
Needs correction within 1 hr |

Ensure ABCs.
Notify Senior Resident. ☎ _____

→ Transfer to ICU.
→ **Seizures**
(See p 142)
→ **Increased ICP**
(See p 134)
Place arterial catheter.

Repeat
nifedipine PO/SL/NG.

sodium nitroprusside IV infusion
or **labetalol** IV infusion
or **nitroglycerin** IV infusion

→ Workup ← **(D)**

✳(Continued from p 150)

Ⓓ **History:** pheochromocytoma (*sweats, fever, palpitations, FTT, weight loss*), CVA/TIA (*transient blindness*), increased ICP (*headache, vomiting*), hyperaldosteronism (*cramps, weakness, constipation*), congenital adrenal hyperplasia, pre-eclampsia (*menarche, LMP*), renal (*polyuria, polydipsia, hematuria, edema*), collagen vascular disease (*joint pain / swelling, edema*)

Family history: hypertension, CVA, renal disease

Neonatal history: umbilical artery/venous catheter

Medications: over-the-counter medications, oral contraceptives, ingestions

Classical findings: Cushingoid (*moon facies, hirsutism, truncal obesity, striae*), Turner's syndrome (*webbed neck, low hairline, widely spaced nipples*), William's syndrome (*elfin facies, poor growth, murmur, hypercalcemia*), fundi (*retinal hemorrhages, cotton-wool exudates, AV nicking*), thyromegaly, cardiac (*gallop, murmur, hyperdynamic*), dyspnea, rales, abdominal bruits or masses

Nephrology consult ☎_____

Ⓔ Capsule may be punctured with a tuberculin syringe, and contents aspirated. May be given sublingually or administered via nasogastric tube, which should then be flushed and clamped for 1 hour.

Table 12-2.   Antihypertensive agents

Agent	Dose	Onset	Duration	Comment
Calcium channel blocker **nifedipine** (Procardia)	0.25-0.5 mg/kg PO/ SL/NG q 15 min then q 3-4 hr	10-30 min	4-6 hr	5 mg cap ≅ 0.175 ml 10 mg cap ≅ 0.35 ml Ⓔ
Arterial/venous vasodilator **sodium nitroprusside** (Nipride)	0.5-8.0 µg/kg/min IV	30 sec	very short	Precise control Watch thiocyanate levels, for methemoglobinemia, and seizures.
Venous vasodilator **nitroglycerin**	1.0-5.0 µg/kg/min IV	immediate	very short	Adjust dose according to renal function.
Alpha/beta blocker **labetalol** (Normodyne)	0.25 mg/kg IV over 1-2 min q 10-15 min 1-3 mg/kg/hr or 0.015-0.05 mg/kg/min	immediate	10 hr	<u>max</u>. 3.25 mg/kg total Use with caution in patients with bradycardia or asthma.

NOTE: In chronic hypertension, lower BP slowly.

Hypernatremia

Maria Asi-Bautista

> Hypernatremic dehydration is usually seen when infants are fed boiled skim milk or homemade electrolyte solutions with high salt content. Infants are at a greater risk for this type of dehydration because of greater water loss secondary to higher body surface area:weight ratio.

(A) Vital signs or evidence of poor perfusion may not appear until 12-18% of weight is lost. If degree of dehydration by history is greater than by physical examination, consider hypernatremic dehydration.

(B) Symptoms usually occur when serum $Na^+ > 160$ mEq/L or osmolality > 340 mOsm/L; may also be associated with hypocalcemia and hyperglycemia.

(C) If $\frac{U}{P}$ osmolality is < 2, DI should be considered. Polyuria will be present and urinalysis will show normal parameters except for a specific gravity < 1.006 or urine osmolality < 200 mOsm/L despite dehydration. CT scan or MRI should be considered to rule out suprasellar mass.

(D) Sample calculation

Weight	7.0 kg	measured serum Na^+	165 mEq/L
% dehydration	10 %	desired serum Na^+	145 mEq/L

TBW (total body water) = (0.6)(weight in kg)

	Maintenance	Replacement	Total[b]
Water	(100 ml/kg/day) (700 ml)(2 days) **= 1400 ml**	(10%)(7.0 kg) **700 ml** Free water deficit[a] 580 ml Remainder, as NS 120 ml	**2100 ml** or **2.1 L** over 48 hours
Na^+	3 mEq/100 ml fluid/day $\frac{3mEq}{100ml} \times \frac{700ml}{1} = 21$ mEq (21 mEq)(2days) **= 42 mEq**	(120 ml)(154mEq/L) (1L/1000 ml)= **18 mEq**	**60 mEq**

[a] Free water deficit

$$\left[\frac{[Na^+]_{measured}}{[Na^+]_{desired}} (TBW) \right] - TBW$$

$$\left[\frac{165}{145} (0.6)(7.0) \right] - (0.6)(7.0) = 580 \text{ ml}$$

[b] $\frac{60 \text{ mEq } Na^+}{2100 \text{ ml}}$ or $\frac{28 \text{ mEq } Na^+}{1000 \text{ ml}}$ or 0.2 NS (approximately)

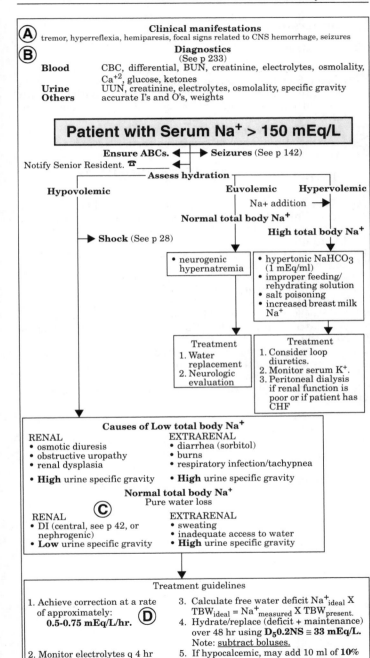

Clinical manifestations

(A) tremor, hyperreflexia, hemiparesis, focal signs related to CNS hemorrhage, seizures

(B) **Diagnostics**
(See p 233)

Blood	CBC, differential, BUN, creatinine, electrolytes, osmolality, Ca^{+2}, glucose, ketones
Urine	UUN, creatinine, electrolytes, osmolality, specific gravity
Others	accurate I's and O's, weights

Patient with Serum Na^+ > 150 mEq/L

Ensure ABCs. ◄──► **Seizures** (See p 142)

Notify Senior Resident. ☎_____

Assess hydration

Hypovolemic   **Euvolemic**   **Hypervolemic**

Na+ addition ──►

Normal total body Na^+

High total body Na^+

► **Shock** (See p 28)

- neurogenic hypernatremia

- hypertonic $NaHCO_3$ (1 mEq/ml)
- improper feeding/ rehydrating solution
- salt poisoning
- increased breast milk Na^+

Treatment
1. Water replacement
2. Neurologic evaluation

Treatment
1. Consider loop diuretics.
2. Monitor serum K^+.
3. Peritoneal dialysis if renal function is poor or if patient has CHF

Causes of Low total body Na^+

RENAL
- osmotic diuresis
- obstructive uropathy
- renal dysplasia
- **High** urine specific gravity

EXTRARENAL
- diarrhea (sorbitol)
- burns
- respiratory infection/tachypnea
- **High** urine specific gravity

Normal total body Na^+
(C) Pure water loss

RENAL
- DI (central, see p 42, or nephrogenic)
- **Low** urine specific gravity

EXTRARENAL
- sweating
- inadequate access to water
- **High** urine specific gravity

Treatment guidelines

1. Achieve correction at a rate of approximately: (D) **0.5-0.75 mEq/L/hr.**

2. Monitor electrolytes q 4 hr and change solution accordingly.

3. Calculate free water deficit Na^+_{ideal} X TBW_{ideal} = $Na^+_{measured}$ X $TBW_{present}$.

4. Hydrate/replace (deficit + maintenance) over 48 hr using **$D_5 0.2NS \cong 33$ mEq/L.** Note: <u>subtract boluses.</u>

5. If hypocalcemic, may add 10 ml of **10%** **Ca^{+2} gluconate** per 500-ml solution.

Hyponatremia

Maria Asi-Bautista

(A) Clinical effects are primarily the result of cerebral edema. Slowly developing hyponatremia is better tolerated than an acute fall in Na^+ level. Most patients with hyponatremia who present in coma have serum $Na^+ < 120$ mEq/L.

(B) Serial labs needed

(C) Artificial reduction of measured serum Na^+, i.e., pseudo-hyponatremia.

$$\text{True Na}^+ = 2Na^+ + \frac{\text{measured Osm-calculated Osm}}{2}$$

(D) True low sodium concentration due to redistribution of intracellular H_2O into the extracellular space. For each 100 mg/dL increase in blood glucose, serum Na^+ decreases by 1.6 mEq/L.

(E) Losses from sweating are sometimes replaced with low-salt or salt-free drinks.

Hyponatremia may be associated with:
metabolic alkalosis → loss of gastric juice
metabolic acidosis → loss of lower GI tract secretions.

(F) Suspect adrenal insufficiency when low serum Na^+ is associated with $U_{Na} > 20$ mEq/L and hyperkalemia which is NOT the result of oliguric renal failure.

(G) Severe symptomatic hyponatremia is most common in this group. Despite increase in water intake, no edema is observed.

(H) History and physical exam usually lead to diagnosis.

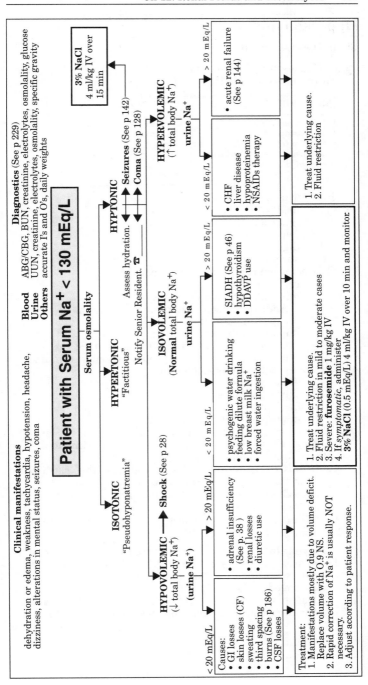

Clinical manifestations
dehydration or edema, weakness, tachycardia, hypotension, headache, dizziness, alterations in mental status, seizures, coma

Diagnostics (See p 229)
Blood ABG/CBG, BUN, creatinine, electrolytes, osmolality, glucose
Urine UUN, creatinine, electrolytes, osmolality, specific gravity
Others accurate I's and O's, daily weights

Patient with Serum Na⁺ < 130 mEq/L

Serum osmolality

HYPERTONIC
"Factitious"

HYPOTONIC
Assess hydration. ☎
Notify Senior Resident.

ISOTONIC
"Pseudohyponatremia"

ISOTONIC → **Shock** (See p 28)

HYPOVOLEMIC (↓ total body Na⁺)
(urine Na⁺)

< 20 mEq/L
Causes:
• GI losses
• skin losses (CF)
• sweating
• third spacing
• burns (See p 186)
• CSF losses

> 20 mEq/L
• adrenal insufficiency (See p. 38)
• renal losses
• diuretic use

Treatment:
1. Manifestations mostly due to volume deficit. Replace volume with 0.9 NS.
2. Rapid correction of Na⁺ is usually NOT necessary.
3. Adjust according to patient response.

ISOVOLEMIC (Normal total body Na⁺)
urine Na⁺

< 20 mEq/L
• psychogenic water drinking
• feeding dilute formula
• low breast milk Na⁺
• forced water ingestion

> 20 mEq/L
• SIADH (See p 46)
• hypothyroidism
• DDAVP use

1. Treat underlying cause.
2. Fluid restriction in mild to moderate cases
3. Severe: **furosemide** 1 mg/kg IV
4. If *symptomatic*, administer **3% NaCl** (0.5 mEq/L) 4 ml/kg IV over 10 min and monitor.

HYPERVOLEMIC (↑ total body Na⁺)
urine Na⁺

< 20 mEq/L
• CHF
• liver disease
• hypoproteinemia
• NSAIDs therapy

> 20 mEq/L
• acute renal failure (See p 144)

1. Treat underlying cause.
2. Fluid restriction

Seizures (See p 142)
Coma (See p 128)

3% NaCl
4 ml/kg IV over 15 min

Hyperkalemia

Silvia Operti-Considine

(A) Causes of hyperkalemia
A. Increased K^+ load

EXOGENOUS	ENDOGENOUS
PO/IV supplements salt substitutes penicillin with K^+ in high doses transfusion with stored blood poisoning	intravascular hemolysis rhabdomyolysis trauma burns tumor lysis starvation

B. Transcellular shift of K^+:
> acidosis
> insulin deficiency
> hyperosmolality
> digoxin overdose
> succinylcholine

C. Decreased renal excretory capacity:
> renal failure
> mineralocorticoid deficiency:
>> Addison's disease, hyperaldosteronism
>> K^+-sparing diuretics
> impaired tubular secretion:
>> sickle cell disease, renal transplant, SLE,
>> obstructive uropathy, pseudohypoaldosteronism

(B) Causes of pseudohyperkalemia:
> leukocytosis
> thrombocytosis
> in vitro hemolysis
> improper collection of blood

(C) These measures will decrease the serum K^+ level by shifting K^+ from the extracellular compartment to the intracellular compartment.

A. **Calcium gluconate 10%:** reduces the cardiotoxic effects of K^+ by membrane stabilization

B. **NaHCO$_3$:** alkalosis will cause K^+ to move from the ECF to the ICF

C. **Glucose/insulin:** insulin also will promote K^+ shift from the ECF to the ICF.

(D) **Kayexalate:** a resin binder that decreases the total K^+ content. Administer PO or PR. When given rectally, it should be retained for 2-3 hours to be effective. 1 mEq K^+ is exchanged with 1 mEq Na^+.

(E) β_2- agonists, e.g., albuterol IV, have been used in adults, but the decrease in K^+ levels has been unpredictable.

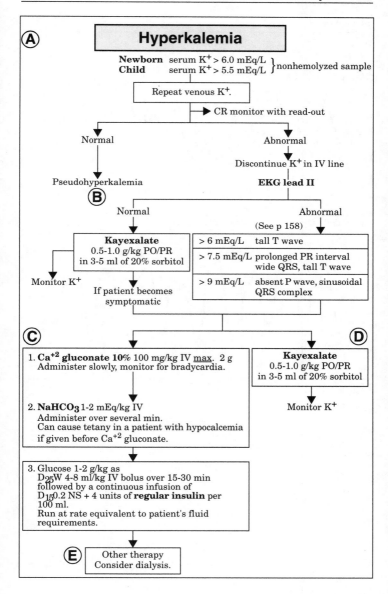

(A) **Hyperkalemia**

Newborn serum K$^+$ > 6.0 mEq/L } nonhemolyzed sample
Child   serum K$^+$ > 5.5 mEq/L

Repeat venous K$^+$.

→ CR monitor with read-out

Normal   Abnormal

                               Discontinue K$^+$ in IV line

Pseudohyperkalemia   **EKG lead II**

(B)

Normal   Abnormal

                               (See p 158)

Kayexalate | > 6 mEq/L | tall T wave |
0.5-1.0 g/kg PO/PR | > 7.5 mEq/L | prolonged PR interval wide QRS, tall T wave |
in 3-5 ml of 20% sorbitol | > 9 mEq/L | absent P wave, sinusoidal QRS complex |

Monitor K$^+$

If patient becomes
symptomatic

(C)   (D)

1. **Ca^{+2} gluconate 10%** 100 mg/kg IV <u>max</u>. 2 g | **Kayexalate**
   Administer slowly, monitor for bradycardia. | 0.5-1.0 g/kg PO/PR
                                                             | in 3-5 ml of 20% sorbitol
                                                             |
                                                             | Monitor K$^+$
2. **NaHCO$_3$** 1-2 mEq/kg IV
   Administer over several min.
   Can cause tetany in a patient with hypocalcemia
   if given before Ca^{+2} gluconate.

3. Glucose 1-2 g/kg as
   D$_{25}$W 4-8 ml/kg IV bolus over 15-30 min
   followed by a continuous infusion of
   D$_{15}$0.2 NS + 4 units of **regular insulin** per
   100 ml.
   Run at rate equivalent to patient's fluid
   requirements.

(E) Other therapy
     Consider dialysis.

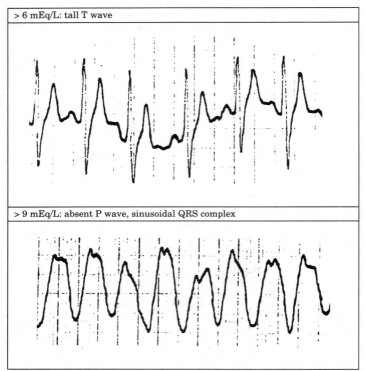

> 6 mEq/L: tall T wave

> 9 mEq/L: absent P wave, sinusoidal QRS complex

Figure 12-1.

Notes

Hypocalcemia

Jolene Ellis

(A) Early onset (during first 3 days of life)

Maternal: diabetes, toxemia, obstetric complications, severe vitamin D deficiency, hyperparathyroidism

Intrapartum: asphyxia, prematurity

Postnatal: hypoxia, shock, asphyxia, RDS, sepsis, bicarbonate therapy, transfusion of citrated blood, hypoparathyroidism

(B) Late onset (after first 3 days of life): any of the causes under **(A)**

Also consider: high phosphate diet, intestinal malabsorption, renal disease, defect in vitamin D metabolism, Mg^{+2} deficiency, DiGeorge syndrome.

(C) Total serum $Ca^{+2} \cong 40\%$ ionized calcium, 50% protein bound, and 10% remains complexed. Ionized values listed are **not** normalized for pH.

(D) 1 ml of **10% Ca^{+2} gluconate** $\cong 100$ mg $\cong 9$ mg of elemental Ca^{+2}.
1 ml of **10% Ca^{+2} chloride** $\cong 100$ mg $\cong 27$ mg of elemental Ca^{+2}.

(E) Maintenance Ca^{+2} is 45-90 mg/kg/day of elemental Ca^{+2}.

(F) A drop in serum albumin of **1 g/dL lowers** serum Ca^{+2} by **0.8 mg/dL**. Correct hypocalcemia before correcting **acidosis**.

Acidosis **increases** ionized Ca^{+2} concentration.
Alkalosis **decreases** ionized Ca^{+2} concentration.

Metastatic calcification may occur when the ion product of serum Ca^{+2} and phosphorus exceeds **60**.

(G) Causes of Mg^{+2} deficiency: familial hypomagnesemia, malabsorption syndromes (short gut syndrome), infants of diabetic mothers

(H) Causes: X-linked recessive trait, DiGeorge syndrome, transient hypofunction or congenital aplasia of the parathyroids, maternal diabetes, maternal alcoholism

(I) Causes: Addison's disease, mucocutaneous candidiasis, hemosiderosis, Wilson's disease (copper deposition)

(J) Causes of vitamin D deficiency: dietary deficiency, malabsorption, altered metabolism, impaired synthesis, renal failure, genetic deficiency of 1-alpha-hydroxylase

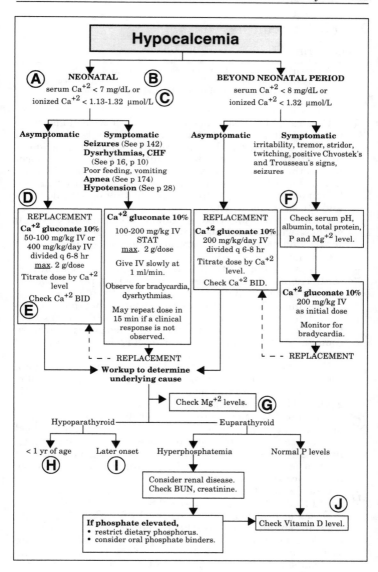

Hypocalcemia

(A) NEONATAL (B)
serum Ca^{+2} < 7 mg/dL or **(C)**
ionized Ca^{+2} < 1.13-1.32 µmol/L

BEYOND NEONATAL PERIOD
serum Ca^{+2} < 8 mg/dL or
ionized Ca^{+2} < 1.32 µmol/L

Asymptomatic

Symptomatic
Seizures (See p 142)
Dysrhythmias, CHF
(See p 16, p 10)
Poor feeding, vomiting
Apnea (See p 174)
Hypotension (See p 28)

Asymptomatic

Symptomatic
irritability, tremor, stridor,
twitching, positive Chvostek's
and Trousseau's signs,
seizures

(D)

REPLACEMENT
Ca^{+2} gluconate 10%
50-100 mg/kg IV or
400 mg/kg/day IV
divided q 6-8 hr
<u>max</u>. 2 g/dose
Titrate dose by Ca^{+2}
level
Check Ca^{+2} BID
(E)

Ca^{+2} gluconate 10%
100-200 mg/kg IV
STAT
<u>max</u>. 2 g/dose

Give IV slowly at
1 ml/min.

Observe for bradycardia,
dysrhythmias.

May repeat dose in
15 min if a clinical
response is not
observed.

REPLACEMENT
Ca^{+2} gluconate 10%
200 mg/kg/day IV
divided q 6-8 hr
Titrate dose by Ca^{+2}
level.
Check Ca^{+2} BID.

(F)

Check serum pH,
albumin, total protein,
P and Mg^{+2} level.

Ca^{+2} gluconate 10%
200 mg/kg IV
as initial dose

Monitor for
bradycardia.

└ ─ ─ REPLACEMENT

└ ─ ─ REPLACEMENT

**Workup to determine
underlying cause**

Check Mg^{+2} levels. **(G)**

Hypoparathyroid ─────── Euparathyroid

< 1 yr of age
(H)

Later onset
(I)

Hyperphosphatemia

Normal P levels

Consider renal disease.
Check BUN, creatinine.

If phosphate elevated,
• restrict dietary phosphorus.
• consider oral phosphate binders.

Check Vitamin D level. **(J)**

Metabolic Acidosis

Sunita Sarin

> A primary decrease in plasma bicarbonate concentration with a
> decrease in serum pH. A biochemical derangement (not a disease)
> that results from a disequilibrium between production and excretion of
> acids.

(A) Generally, metabolic acidosis presents with nonspecific findings. Often the underlying cause is reflected in clinical manifestations. Consider the presence of metabolic acidosis in a patient who exhibits Kussmaul breathing or is hyperpneic in the absence of obvious lung pathology. Keep in mind the variety of underlying causes which can be divided into two main groups: (1) increased production of organic acids and (2) loss of bicarbonate.

Children with inherited metabolic abnormalities as well as those with renal disease may have FTT. Consider toxins, sepsis, and necrotizing enterocolitis in cases of unexplained metabolic acidosis.

(B) Serum pH and electrolyte concentrations are both important. The blood gas will reveal a low serum pH with a low calculated bicarbonate, while the electrolytes will reveal a low serum CO_2. In acute uncompensated metabolic acidosis, each increase in $PaCO_2$ of 10 mmHg will decrease pH by 0.8. In cases of chronic metabolic acidosis, respiratory compensation (hyperventilation) occurs in 1-2 hours and renal compensation in 24 hours.

Other laboratory tests may be indicated: osmolal gap, comprehensive drug screen (include alcohols), metabolic, amino acid and organic acid screens, sepsis workup, lactic acid, EKG rhythm strip.

(C) The most common cause of metabolic acidosis is hypovolemia, and thus can be corrected by restoration of blood volume, cardiac output, and improved tissue perfusion. An important consideration in children is a lack of sustained respiratory compensation, therefore, early ventilatory assistance should be provided.

(D) Calculation of bicarbonate deficit = (desired HCO_3 - measured HCO_3) X weight (in kg) X 0.6 bicarbonate deficit

Doses of bicarbonate in excess of 1.0 mEq/kg/dose may lead to an alkaline overshoot and should therefore be avoided. For each 0.1 increase in pH, O_2 availability to the tissues may decrease by 10% secondary to a shift in the oxyhemoglobin dissociation curve to the left. Monitor arterial PaO_2 and O_2 saturations.

✱(Continued on p 166)

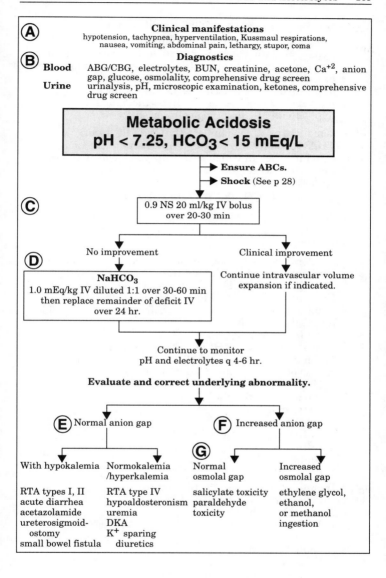

(A) **Clinical manifestations**
hypotension, tachypnea, hyperventilation, Kussmaul respirations,
nausea, vomiting, abdominal pain, lethargy, stupor, coma

(B) **Diagnostics**
Blood   ABG/CBG, electrolytes, BUN, creatinine, acetone, Ca^{+2}, anion
            gap, glucose, osmolality, comprehensive drug screen
Urine   urinalysis, pH, microscopic examination, ketones, comprehensive
            drug screen

Metabolic Acidosis
pH < 7.25, HCO$_3$ < 15 mEq/L

➤ **Ensure ABCs.**
➤ **Shock** (See p 28)

(C) 0.9 NS 20 ml/kg IV bolus
over 20-30 min

No improvement   Clinical improvement

(D) **NaHCO$_3$**
1.0 mEq/kg IV diluted 1:1 over 30-60 min
then replace remainder of deficit IV
over 24 hr.

Continue intravascular volume
expansion if indicated.

Continue to monitor
pH and electrolytes q 4-6 hr.

Evaluate and correct underlying abnormality.

(E) Normal anion gap   **(F)** Increased anion gap

(G)

With hypokalemia   Normokalemia   Normal   Increased
                   /hyperkalemia   osmolal gap   osmolal gap

RTA types I, II   RTA type IV   salicylate toxicity   ethylene glycol,
acute diarrhea   hypoaldosteronism paraldehyde   ethanol,
acetazolamide   uremia   toxicity   or methanol
ureterosigmoid-   DKA   ingestion
    ostomy   K$^+$ sparing
small bowel fistula   diuretics

✳(Continued from p 164)

Other complications of bicarbonate therapy:
- hyperosmolality/hypernatremia in premature infants and newborns; may result in intracranial hemorrhage
- paradoxical CSF acidosis
hypercarbia: $NaHCO_3 \longleftrightarrow Na^+ + H_2O + CO_2$
- may aggravate pre-existing hypocalcemia and hypokalemia by inducing cellular shifts

Other therapeutic modalities that may be used:
- THAM (tris-hydroxy-methyl-amino-methane) is indicated in cases in which respiratory acidosis (CO_2) retention is a concern. May cause respiratory depression, hyperkalemia and hypoglycemia.

$THAM + H_3CO_3 \longleftrightarrow THAM-H+ + HCO_3^-$

$$\updownarrow$$

$$CO_2 + H_2O$$

- dichloroacetate for severe lactic acidosis
- carbicarb: an equimolar solution of $NaHCO_3$ and Na_2CO_3. Does not lead to increased CO_2 levels
Currently under study in human subjects
- hemodialysis/peritoneal dialysis for severe intractable metabolic acidosis

 Calculation of anion gap =
  $[Na^+ + K^+] - [Cl^- + HCO_3^-]$ Normal values 12-16
Normal anion gap metabolic acidosis is primarily caused by a loss of bicarbonate. Causes include:
  Ureteroenterostomy   (USED CARP)
  Small bowel fistula
  Extra chloride
  Diarrhea
  Carbonic anhydrase inhibitors
  Adrenal insufficiency
  Renal tubular acidosis
  Pancreatic fistula.

Ⓕ Increased anion gap (> 16) metabolic acidosis is caused by the increased production of organic acids.
Causes include the following:
  Methanol   (MUD PILES)
  Uremia
  Diabetic ketoacidosis
  Paraldehyde
  Iron/isoniazid/inhalants (cyanide, CO)
  Lactic acidosis
  Ethanol/ethylene glycol
  Salicylates, starvation, solvents (toluene).

(G) Calculation of osmolal gap = measured osmolality - calculated osmolality

Normal value < 10

Calculated osmolality (mOsm/L) =

$$2\ [\ Na^+]\ (mEq/L) + \frac{BUN\ (mg/dL)}{2.8} + \frac{glucose\ (mg/dL)}{18}$$

Respiratory

Acute Bronchiolitis

Mary Lieh-Lai

> Acute bronchiolitis is a clinical syndrome of expiratory wheezing and
> hyperexpansion of the lungs on chest radiograph in children < 6
> months.

(A) Usually affects infants < 6 months of age during the months of October through April. URI symptoms are prominent with copious nasal discharge.

(B)

	RSV nasal wash
Materials	sterile ear syringe
	medicine cup
	3-5 ml sterile saline
	sterile tube

Place child in upright position. Dispense 3-5 ml of sterile saline into medicine cup. Draw saline into ear syringe. Incline patient's head backward at about 70° angle. Occlude nostril with a gloved finger. Insert ear syringe into other nostril, squirt saline, and immediately re-aspirate. Remove syringe from nostril and empty into sterile tube. Submit to laboratory.

(C) The benefits of the use of theophylline and steroids have not been shown.

(D) High risk patients (1994 Red Book recommendations)
- hospitalized infants ≤ 6 weeks of age
- children with multiple congenital anomalies or certain neurologic diseases, e.g., severe CP, MG
- patients undergoing chemotherapy for malignancy
- recent transplant recipient
- premature infants
- immunocompromised children, especially those with AIDS or SCID.
- children with complicated CHD
- Children with bronchopulmonary dysplasia, CF, or other chronic lung conditions
- severely ill infants, i.e., PaO_2 < 65 mmHg with increasing $PaCO_2$
- all mechanically ventilated patients with RSV infection

(E) **Ribavirin** is teratogenic and mutagenic in small animals and has been demonstrated to cross the placenta. However, these effects have not been shown in humans.

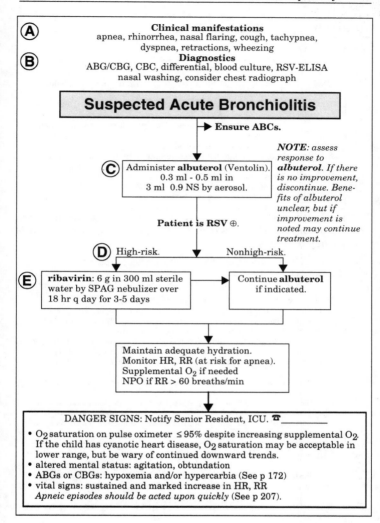

(A)
Clinical manifestations
apnea, rhinorrhea, nasal flaring, cough, tachypnea,
dyspnea, retractions, wheezing
(B)
Diagnostics
ABG/CBG, CBC, differential, blood culture, RSV-ELISA
nasal washing, consider chest radiograph

Suspected Acute Bronchiolitis

➤ **Ensure ABCs.**

(C) Administer **albuterol** (Ventolin).
0.3 ml - 0.5 ml in
3 ml 0.9 NS by aerosol.

*NOTE: assess
response to
albuterol. If there
is no improvement,
discontinue. Bene-
fits of albuterol
unclear, but if
improvement is
noted may continue
treatment.*

Patient is RSV ⊕.

(D) High-risk.   Nonhigh-risk.

(E) **ribavirin**: 6 g in 300 ml sterile
water by SPAG nebulizer over
18 hr q day for 3-5 days   →   Continue **albuterol**
if indicated.

Maintain adequate hydration.
Monitor HR, RR (at risk for apnea).
Supplemental O_2 if needed
NPO if RR > 60 breaths/min

DANGER SIGNS: Notify Senior Resident, ICU. ☎_____

• O_2 saturation on pulse oximeter ≤95% despite increasing supplemental O_2.
If the child has cyanotic heart disease, O_2 saturation may be acceptable in
lower range, but be wary of continued downward trends.
• altered mental status: agitation, obtundation
• ABGs or CBGs: hypoxemia and/or hypercarbia (See p 172)
• vital signs: sustained and marked increase in HR, RR
Apneic episodes should be acted upon quickly (See p 207).

Acute Respiratory Failure

Mary Lieh-Lai

	Causes of acute respiratory failure (partial list)	
CNS	Increased ICP: obstructed shunt, brain tumor, head trauma, etc.	
	Depressant drugs: morphine, midazolam, lorazepam, phenobarbital	
	Neuromuscular disease: Guillain-Barré, MG, status epilepticus	
	Infections: meningitis, encephalitis	
AIRWAY	croup, epiglottitis, asthma, bronchiolitis, foreign body, subglottic stenosis, tonsillar/adenoidal hypertrophy	
PARENCHYMAL/PLEURAL DISEASE		
	pneumonia, pneumothorax, hemothorax	
OTHERS	shock, CHF, sepsis, toxins	

Patients with neuromuscular disease may be in overt respiratory failure without manifesting signs of respiratory distress.

Ⓑ ABG/CBG may show hypoxemia ± hypercarbia.

Ⓒ
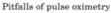

Pitfalls of pulse oximetry
There may be an inherent inaccuracy of up to 4%.
1. Determined by the oxyhemoglobin dissociation curve. The curve flattens with PaO_2 >70 mmHg, therefore, large changes in PaO_2 will result in only small changes in pulse oximeter recording.
2. Presence of abnormal hemoglobin such as COHb or metHb will lead to overestimations of O_2 saturation, because the pulse oximeter only detects saturated and unsaturated Hb, not what the Hb is saturated with.
3. Conditions with peripheral vasoconstriction and decreased pulsatile flow can lead to inaccurate readings.
4. *If the pulse oximeter alarms frequently, determine the cause instead of turning the machine off; a patient may be in shock, and with decreased peripheral perfusion, the pulse oximeter cannot detect pulsatile flow, setting off the alarm.*

Ⓓ Maximum O_2 is delivered only with proper administration.

Ⓔ **Naloxone** is indicated for respiratory depression caused by drugs such as **morphine** and **fentanyl.**

Ⓕ Repeated doses of **flumazenil** have been known to precipitate seizures.

Clinical manifestations

(A) tachycardia, tachypnea, apnea, hypoventilation, decreased air entry, poor or absent respiratory effort, increased retractions, agitation, air hunger, lethargy, obtundation

Diagnostics

(B) **Blood**   ABG/CBG, CBC, differential, BUN, creatinine, electrolytes, osmolality, glucose, consider comprehensive drug screen
Urine   urinalysis, osmolality, comprehensive drug screen
Imaging   chest radiograph, lateral neck (if applicable)

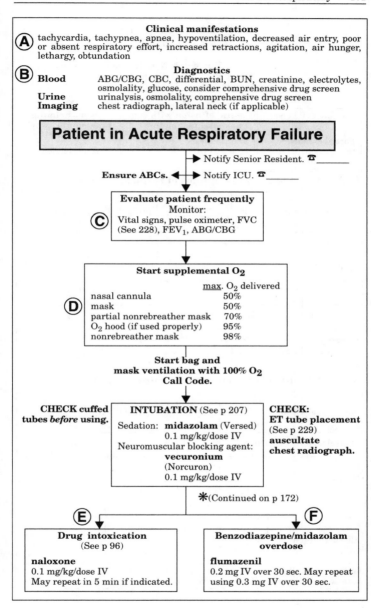

Patient in Acute Respiratory Failure

➤ Notify Senior Resident. ☎_____

Ensure ABCs. ◄— ➤ Notify ICU. ☎_____

Evaluate patient frequently
Monitor:
(C) Vital signs, pulse oximeter, FVC
(See 228), FEV$_1$, ABG/CBG

Start supplemental O$_2$

	max. O$_2$ delivered
nasal cannula	50%
mask	50%
partial nonrebreather mask	70%
O$_2$ hood (if used properly)	95%
nonrebreather mask	98%

(D)

**Start bag and
mask ventilation with 100% O$_2$
Call Code.**

**CHECK cuffed
tubes *before* using.**

INTUBATION (See p 207)

Sedation: **midazolam** (Versed)
0.1 mg/kg/dose IV
Neuromuscular blocking agent:
vecuronium
(Norcuron)
0.1 mg/kg/dose IV

**CHECK:
ET tube placement**
(See p 229)
**auscultate
chest radiograph.**

✱(Continued on p 172)

(E)

Drug intoxication
(See p 96)

naloxone
0.1 mg/kg/dose IV
May repeat in 5 min if indicated.

(F)

**Benzodiazepine/midazolam
overdose**

flumazenil
0.2 mg IV over 30 sec. May repeat
using 0.3 mg IV over 30 sec.

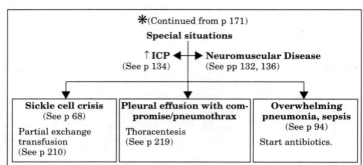

✴(Continued from p 171)

Special situations

↑ICP ◄────► Neuromuscular Disease
(See p 134)   (See pp 132, 136)

Sickle cell crisis (See p 68) Partial exchange transfusion (See p 210)	**Pleural effusion with compromise/pneumothrax** Thoracentesis (See p 219)	**Overwhelming pneumonia, sepsis** (See p 94) Start antibiotics.

Table 13-1. Signs and symptoms of respiratory disease

Symptoms	Extrathoracic	Intrathoracic/ extrapulmonary	Intrapulmonary	Parenchymal
Tachypnea	-	+	+	++++
Stridor	++++	-	-	-
Grunting	-	-	-	++++
Retractions	++++	++	++	++
Wheezing	-	++	++++	-

Table 13-2. Blood gases in acute respiratory failure

Site of involvement		pH	PaCO$_2$	PaO$_2$	Response to 100% O$_2$
Central airway obstruction		↓	↑↑	↓↓	excellent
Peripheral airway obstruction	mild	↑	↓	↓	excellent
	moderate	↔	↔	↓↓	good
	severe	↓	↑	↓↓↓	fair
Alveolar/interstitial pathology	fatigue	↓	↑	↓↓↓	poor

(Tables 13-1 and 13-2) Ashok P. Sarnaik, MD, Chief, Division of
Critical Care Medicine, Children's Hospital of Michigan

Notes

Apnea

Mary Lieh-Lai

> Apnea is defined as the cessation of breathing lasting for > 15 seconds or less if associated with color changes and/or bradycardia.

(A) **Apparent life-threatening event (ALTE):** an episode that is frightening to the observer and is characterized by a combination of apnea (central or occasionally obstructive), color change (usually cyanosis or pallor but occasionally, erythema or plethora), marked change in muscle tone (usually limp), choking or gagging.

Periodic breathing: a breathing pattern in which there are three or more respiratory pauses of greater than 3 seconds duration with less than 20 seconds of respiration between pauses. Periodic breathing may be a normal event.

(B) **Central apnea:** is characterized by the lack of initiation of breathing. Other causes include: RSV infection, central hypoventilation syndrome, prematurity, SCI, head injury, severe anemia, hypoxia, drug ingestion, and metabolic disorders.

(C) **Obstructive apnea:** is caused by airway obstruction that leads to increased resistance and poor to no ventilation despite adequate respiratory effort. Other causes include tonsillar and adenoidal enlargement, gastroesophageal reflux, and vascular ring.

Clinical manifestations

tachycardia, bradycardia, cyanosis, pallor, may be associated with stridor and wheezing (obstructive apnea), findings generally depend on site of obstruction

Diagnostics

ABG/CBG, CBC, differential, BUN, creatinine, electrolytes, glucose, comprehensive urine and serum drug screen, RSV-ELISA nasal washing, sepsis workup, chest and lateral neck radiographs

Consider: CT scan of head, magnified airway radiographs, esophagogram, scintiscan, EKG, EEG, metabolic screen.

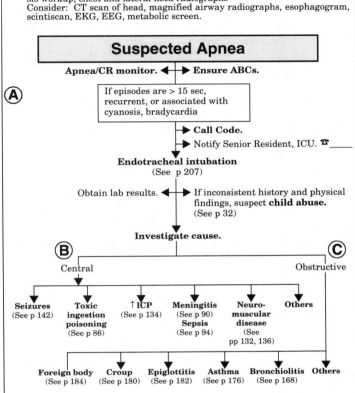

Suspected Apnea

Apnea/CR monitor. ◄──► **Ensure ABCs.**

(A)

If episodes are > 15 sec, recurrent, or associated with cyanosis, bradycardia

► **Call Code.**

► Notify Senior Resident, ICU. ☎ _____

Endotracheal intubation
(See p 207)

Obtain lab results. ◄──► If inconsistent history and physical findings, suspect **child abuse.**
(See p 32)

Investigate cause.

(B) Central   (C) Obstructive

Seizures
(See p 142)

Toxic ingestion poisoning
(See p 86)

↑**ICP**
(See p 134)

Meningitis
(See p 90)
Sepsis
(See p 94)

Neuromuscular disease
(See pp 132, 136)

Others

Foreign body
(See p 184)

Croup
(See p 180)

Epiglottitis
(See p 182)

Asthma
(See p 176)

Bronchiolitis
(See p 168)

Others

Asthma

Alexandre Rotta

> Airflow limitation resulting from a combination of inflammation and obstructive processes that include mucosal edema, bronchospasm, and mucous plugging. Significant air-trapping may lead to pneumothoraces and pneumomediastinum.

(A) If the decision has been made to use **aminophylline**, administer bolus as follows:

if previously on oral theophylline: 3 mg/kg IV as aminophylline
if **not** previously on theophylline: 6 mg/kg IV as aminophylline
1 mg/kg IV aminophylline increases serum level by **2** µg/ml
Check post-bolus level.

theophylline infusion

Age	Dose (mg/kg/hr)
2- 6 mos	0.4
6-11 mos	0.7
1- 9 yr	0.9
9-12 yr	0.7
> 12 yr	0.5

Adjust dose of theophylline in the presence of:
CHF
RSV infection
liver dysfunction
concomitant use of erythromycin,
    cimetidine, or propranolol.
Be wary of theophylline toxicity (See p 124)

methylprednisolone   2 mg/kg IV loading dose
                        1 mg/kg IV q 6 hr maintenance
                        dose

(B) Evaluate all clinical data. Do not base assessment purely on presence or absence of wheezing. Evaluate mental status.

Table 13-3.

Signs and symptoms	Mild	Moderate	Severe
Respiratory rate	30% above mean	30-50% above mean	> 50% above mean
Alertness	normal	normal	decreased
Dyspnea	mild	moderate	severe
Color	good	pale	may be cyanotic
Pulsus paradoxus	< 10 mmHg	10-20 mmHg	20-40 mmHg
Accessory muscle use	mild	moderate	severe
Auscultation	end-exp wheeze	exp, insp wheeze	inaudible wheeze
O_2 saturation	> 95%	90-95%	< 90%
$PaCO_2$	< 35 mmHg	< 40 mmHg	> 40 mmHg
PEFR (predicted)	70-90%	50-70%	< 50%

Modified from *Guidelines for the Diagnosis and Management of Asthma.* National Heart, Lung, and Blood Institute, NIH, Bethesda, Maryland, 9/ 1991, p 105. With permission.

(C) **Table 13-4. Careful monitoring of $PaCO_2$ and O_2 saturation**

	pH	$PaCO_2$	PaO_2
Mild	↑	↓	↓
Moderate	↔	↔	↓↓
Severe	↓	↑	↓↓↓

*(Continued on p 178)

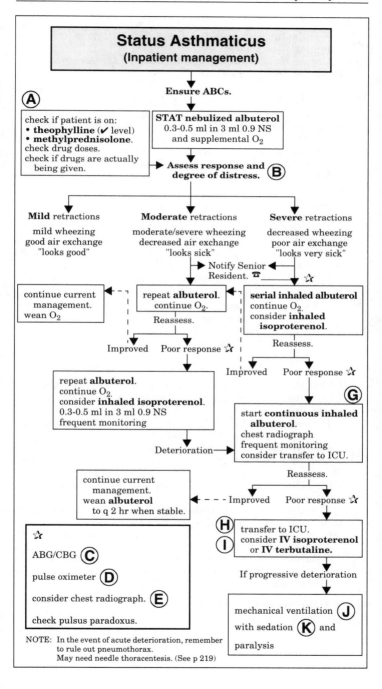

Status Asthmaticus
(Inpatient management)

Ensure ABCs.

(A)
check if patient is on:
- **theophylline** (✔ level)
- **methylprednisolone**.
check drug doses.
check if drugs are actually being given.

STAT nebulized albuterol
0.3-0.5 ml in 3 ml 0.9 NS
and supplemental O_2

Assess response and degree of distress. (B)

Mild retractions

mild wheezing
good air exchange
"looks good"

Moderate retractions

moderate/severe wheezing
decreased air exchange
"looks sick"

Severe retractions

decreased wheezing
poor air exchange
"looks very sick"

Notify Senior Resident. ☎____ ☆

continue current management.
wean O_2

repeat **albuterol**.
continue O_2.
Reassess.

serial inhaled albuterol
continue O_2.
consider **inhaled isoproterenol**.

Reassess.

Improved   Poor response ☆

Improved   Poor response ☆

repeat **albuterol**.
continue O_2.
consider **inhaled isoproterenol**.
0.3-0.5 ml in 3 ml 0.9 NS
frequent monitoring

Deterioration

(G)
start **continuous inhaled albuterol**.
chest radiograph
frequent monitoring
consider transfer to ICU.

Reassess.

continue current management.
wean **albuterol**
to q 2 hr when stable.

Improved   Poor response ☆

(H) transfer to ICU.
(I) consider **IV isoproterenol** or **IV terbutaline**.

If progressive deterioration

☆

ABG/CBG **(C)**

pulse oximeter **(D)**

consider chest radiograph. **(E)**

check pulsus paradoxus.

NOTE: In the event of acute deterioration, remember to rule out pneumothorax.
May need needle thoracentesis. (See p 219)

mechanical ventilation **(J)**
with sedation **(K)** and
paralysis

*(Continued from p 176)

(D) Keep saturation > 95%. Know limitations of the pulse oximeter. (See p 170).

(E) Obtain a chest radiograph if pneumonia, pneumothorax, or foreign body is suspected.

(F) Pulsus paradoxus: exaggerated decrease in systolic BP > 10 mmHg during inspiration due to the following:
- increased blood return to the right ventricle causing septum to bulge into the left ventricle and decrease stroke volume
- increased afterload during inspiration
- exaggerated flattening of the diaphragm causing elongation of the mediastinum and decrease in left ventricular size

Magnitude of pulsus paradoxus correlates with severity of asthma.

Directions: inflate BP cuff above systolic pressure. Deflate slowly. Note pressure at which some heart sounds are heard (expiration). Continue to deflate cuff, and note pressure at which all heart sounds are heard (inspiration). The difference between the two is pulsus paradoxus.

(G) **Continuous albuterol** 0.15-0.45 mg/kg/hr (max. 15 mg/hr)

Example: patient weight = 10 kg
dose desired = 0.15 mg/kg/hr
volume delivered = 10 ml/hr

$$\frac{(10\ kg)(0.15\ mg/kg/hr)}{10\ ml/hr} = \frac{x}{250\ ml} \quad \text{thus}\ x = 37.5\ mg$$

Order as: 38 mg in 250 ml 0.9 NS.

Prolonged use leads to receptor down-regulation. Consider switching to intermittent dosing whenever possible.

Patients should be examined q 4 hr or more frequently. Albuterol infusion should be reordered q 8 hr.

(H) **Continuous IV isoproterenol** 0.05-0.5 µg/kg/min. Titrate dose according to response. Mix 1.0 mg in 100 ml D_5W to obtain 10 µg/ml. (See p 231) Monitor EKG and CPK-MB during infusion. IV isoproterenol should only be used in the ICU setting.

(I) **Continuous IV terbutaline:** administer 2.0 µg/kg IV over 5 min, followed by 4.5 µg/kg/hr IV infusion. In patients receiving theophylline or aminophylline, reduce infusion to 2.25 µg/kg/hr.

(J) Relatively slower rates and larger tidal volumes are recommended. Allow sufficient exhalation time on I:E ratio.

(K) **Midazolam** preferred. 0.05-0.2 mg/kg IV.

(L) **Vecuronium** (Norcuron) 0.1 mg/kg IV.

Notes

Patient with Suspected Croup

Mary Lieh-Lai

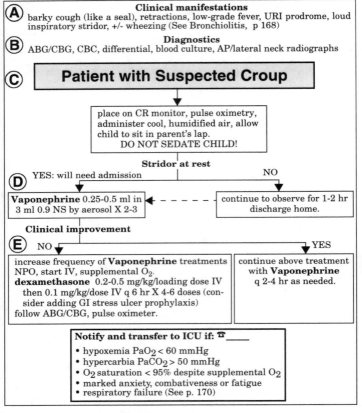

(A) **Clinical manifestations**
barky cough (like a seal), retractions, low-grade fever, URI prodrome, loud inspiratory stridor, +/- wheezing (See Bronchiolitis, p 168)

(B) **Diagnostics**
ABG/CBG, CBC, differential, blood culture, AP/lateral neck radiographs

(C) **Patient with Suspected Croup**

place on CR monitor, pulse oximetry, administer cool, humidified air, allow child to sit in parent's lap.
DO NOT SEDATE CHILD!

Stridor at rest

(D) YES: will need admission   NO

Vaponephrine 0.25-0.5 ml in 3 ml 0.9 NS by aerosol X 2-3 ← — — — — continue to observe for 1-2 hr discharge home.

Clinical improvement

(E) NO   YES

increase frequency of **Vaponephrine** treatments NPO, start IV, supplemental O_2.
dexamethasone 0.2-0.5 mg/kg/loading dose IV then 0.1 mg/kg/dose IV q 6 hr X 4-6 doses (consider adding GI stress ulcer prophylaxis)
follow ABG/CBG, pulse oximeter.

continue above treatment with **Vaponephrine** q 2-4 hr as needed.

Notify and transfer to ICU if: ☎ _____
• hypoxemia $PaO_2 < 60$ mmHg
• hypercarbia $PaCO_2 > 50$ mmHg
• O_2 saturation < 95% despite supplemental O_2
• marked anxiety, combativeness or fatigue
• respiratory failure (See p. 170)

(A) Other signs and symptoms:
6 mos - 3 yr, gradual onset, typically 2-3 day history of URI symptoms
Etiology: viral - parainfluenzae, influenzae, RSV
Differential diagnosis: epiglottitis, vocal cord paralysis, iatrogenic subglottic stenosis or edema (postextubation or postinstrumentation), laryngeal web, foreign body, bacterial tracheitis, retropharyngeal abscess, caustic ingestion

(B) Radiographic findings: "steeple sign" narrowing of trachea because of intraluminal edema

(C) If the patient has a history of recurrent croup, BPD or prior intubation, consider notifying ENT. ☎ _____

(D) Monitor heart rate.

(E) Consider **HeliOx** (to decrease turbulent flow) or **albuterol** (if patient is wheezing). Consider **nebulized budesonide**.

Dislodged Tracheostomy Tube

Mary Lieh-Lai

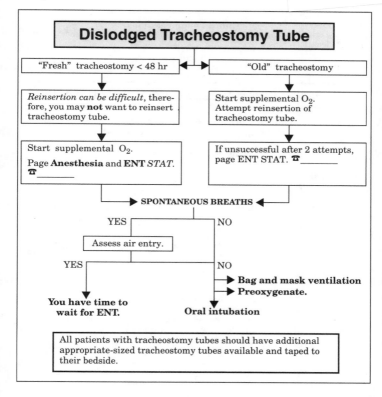

All patients with tracheostomy tubes should have additional appropriate-sized tracheostomy tubes available and taped to their bedside.

piglottitis

Mary Lieh-Lai

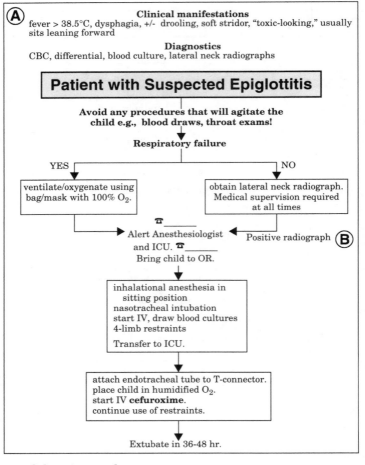

(A) **Clinical manifestations**
fever > 38.5°C, dysphagia, +/- drooling, soft stridor, "toxic-looking," usually sits leaning forward

Diagnostics
CBC, differential, blood culture, lateral neck radiographs

Patient with Suspected Epiglottitis

Avoid any procedures that will agitate the child e.g., blood draws, throat exams!

Respiratory failure

YES — ventilate/oxygenate using bag/mask with 100% O_2.

NO — obtain lateral neck radiograph. Medical supervision required at all times

☎_____
Alert Anesthesiologist and ICU. ☎_____
Bring child to OR.

Positive radiograph **(B)**

inhalational anesthesia in sitting position
nasotracheal intubation
start IV, draw blood cultures
4-limb restraints

Transfer to ICU.

attach endotracheal tube to T-connector.
place child in humidified O_2.
start IV **cefuroxime**.
continue use of restraints.

Extubate in 36-48 hr.

(A) Other signs and symptoms:
typically 2-6 years old, but this pattern is changing to include younger children; acute onset within 8-12 hr

Etiology: *Hemophilus influenzae* in 99% of cases

Differential diagnosis:
croup, bacterial tracheitis, retropharyngeal abscess, angioneurotic edema

(B) Radiographic findings:
enlarged epiglottis and aryepiglottic folds

Notes

Foreign Body Aspiration

Mary Lieh-Lai

> Foreign body aspiration usually occurs in toddlers 1-3 years of age. Less than 30% of children come to medical attention within the first 24 hours. Unless the foreign body is causing complete airway obstruction, initial symptoms may subside.

(A) Signs and symptoms depend on the location of the foreign body. The most common substance aspirated is organic material, especially peanuts. This frequently causes a reactive pneumonitis and fever.

(B) Radiopaque foreign bodies will be visible on chest or lateral neck radiographs. When a radiolucent foreign body is lodged in a mainstem bronchus, a ball-valve phenomenon produces differential expansion secondary to air trapping on the obstructed side. This can be detected by inspiratory/expiratory chest radiographs or by bilateral lateral decubitus films (down side simulates expiration on the affected side). With complete bronchial occlusion, atelectasis is a frequent finding.

ABG/CBG will show hypercarbia, hypoxemia, or both, depending on the site of obstruction.

(C) If antibiotics are indicated, provide coverage for anaerobic organisms. Occasionally, intense inflammation secondary to organic material aspiration may be present, and steroids can be beneficial.

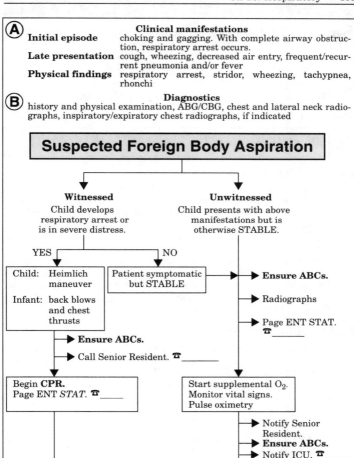

(A) **Clinical manifestations**

Initial episode   choking and gagging. With complete airway obstruction, respiratory arrest occurs.

Late presentation   cough, wheezing, decreased air entry, frequent/recurrent pneumonia and/or fever

Physical findings   respiratory arrest, stridor, wheezing, tachypnea, rhonchi

(B) **Diagnostics**

history and physical examination, ABG/CBG, chest and lateral neck radiographs, inspiratory/expiratory chest radiographs, if indicated

Suspected Foreign Body Aspiration

Witnessed
Child develops respiratory arrest or is in severe distress.

Unwitnessed
Child presents with above manifestations but is otherwise STABLE.

YES   NO

Child: Heimlich maneuver

Infant: back blows and chest thrusts

Patient symptomatic but STABLE

➤ **Ensure ABCs.**

➤ Radiographs

➤ Page ENT STAT. ☎_____

➤ **Ensure ABCs.**

➤ Call Senior Resident. ☎_____

Begin **CPR.**
Page ENT *STAT.* ☎_____

Start supplemental O$_2$.
Monitor vital signs.
Pulse oximetry

➤ Notify Senior Resident.

➤ **Ensure ABCs.**

➤ Notify ICU. ☎_____

(C)
To OR for endoscopic removal

Smoke Inhalation and Surface Burns

Burns: Thermal, Chemical, Electrical

Mary Lieh-Lai and Michelle Rotta

> An injury to tissue resulting from direct thermal insult, exposure to caustic chemicals or radiation, or contact with an electrical current

Partial-thickness burns

First degree: epidermis only; erythema, pain, minimal edema, skin function intact

Second degree (superficial): epidermal destruction plus < 1/2 of dermis; pain, edema with blisters, superficial dermal capillary network still intact, heals in 7-14 days with minimal scarring

Second-degree (deep): epidermal destruction plus > 1/2 of dermis; white leathery marble-like appearance, dry, speckled pattern seen secondary to thrombosed vessels, +/- pain, re-epithelializes slowly. Dense scarring occurs if skin is allowed to heal primarily

Full-thickness burns

Third degree: destruction of epidermis and dermis, pale or charred, avascular and painless; eschar formation secondary to coagulation of dead skin

Fourth degree: above plus fascia, muscle or bone involvement

Admission criteria

1. Partial-thickness burn > 8% BSAB in m^2 or full-thickness burn > 2% BSAB in m^2
2. Burn areas with high risk for disability or poor cosmetic outcome (>1% BSAB of face, perineum, hands, feet, circumferential burns, burns overlying joints)
3. Chemical or electrical burns
4. Presence of associated injuries
5. Suspected child abuse:

   - burns: when the burn pattern does not match the history given
   - submersion injuries: well demarcated, symmetrical or circumferential burns of the buttocks, hands, or feet
   - scalds: absence of splattered or splash pattern
   - cigarette burns: small, deep, circular
   - contact burns: deep, geometric pattern, sharply demarcated borders

✻(Continued on p 188)

(A) **Clinical manifestations**
Determine degree of burn; capillary refill. Note other related trauma. 10% of burn injuries are due to abuse. Look for signs/symptoms of **smoke inhalation/CO poisoning** (See p 190).

Diagnostics

Blood	ABG/CBG, COHb, CBC, differential, electrolytes, BUN, creatinine, Ca^{+2}, glucose, comprehensive serum drug screen, CPK (MB, BB) in electrical burns or soft tissue injury
Urine	urinalysis +/- myoglobin/Hb. Consider comprehensive urine drug screen.
Imaging	chest radiograph. Consider C-spine radiograph.

Suspected Thermal, Chemical, or Electrical Injury

(B)

Stop the burning process

- Remove all clothing.
- Copious irrigation of chemical burns (<u>min</u>. 20 min for chemical eye injuries)
- Remove all jewelry (rings, bracelets, watchbands).

➤ **Ensure ABCs. Stabilize C-spine.**

➤ **100% O_2,**
  CR monitor, Pulse oximeter

➤ Notify Senior Resident. ☎_____
  Notify General Surgery. ☎_____
  Consult Social Services.

With hypovolemia,
administer 20 ml/kg IV **LR.**

First 24 hr, LR solution:

5000 ml/m^2 BSAB/24 hr (burn-related losses)
plus
2000 ml/m^2 BSA/24 hr (maintenance)

May require
escharotomy

(C) Frequent assessment ◄— ➤ NGT **(E)**
of peripheral pulses

(D) Watch for ventilatory limitation secondary to circumferential thorax burns ◄— ➤ Bladder catheter **(F)**

➤ Analgesics **(G)**

Initial wound care

(H)

THERMAL	**ELECTRICAL**
Cover with clean, dry sheet to prevent air contact (decreases pain).	May cause extensive internal injury (more severe than it may appear).
Topical antibiotics: **silver sulfadiazine** (Silvadene) **bacitracin** **povidone iodine** (Betadine)	Look for small depressed entry wound and blown-out exit wound. Dysrhythmias may occur up to 24 hr after injury.
Broad-spectrum antibiotics are usually NOT indicated.	Patients require continuous cardiac monitoring.

CHEMICAL

Once clothing is removed, rinse with copious amounts of sterile water or 0.9 NS. Powdered chemicals should be brushed from skin before flushing.
Chemical eye injuries require a <u>min</u>. of 20 min of continuous irrigation.

✳(Continued from 186)

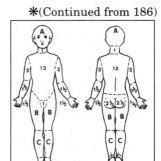

Table 14-1. Percentage of surface area of head and legs at various ages

Area in Diagram	Age in years				
	0	1	5	10	15
A=1/2 of head	9-1/2	8-1/2	6-1/2	5-1/2	4-1/2
B=1/2 of one thigh	2-3/4	3-1/4	4	4-1/4	4-1/2
C=1/2 of one lower leg	2-1/2	2-1/2	2-3/4	3	3-1/4

Solomon JR, Pediatric burns. Crit Card Clin, 1:161, 1985.
With Permission

(A) Pertinent history: did the injury occur in a closed space? Were hazardous chemicals involved? Was the patient intoxicated? Check tetanus immunization status. A history of pre-existing cardiac or renal disease has significant implications in electrical burns and in patients with potential myoglobinuria.

(B) Intubate if there are signs of airway obstruction or if level of consciousness is depressed. (See p 190 for inhalation injury.) IV access may be obtained using aseptic technique in burned areas; avoid circumferential taping.

(C) Edema under the eschar causes decreased venous return, later causing decreased arterial blood flow, ischemia, and gangrene.
- signs of decreased venous return: numbness, pain, cyanosis, weak/absent pulse
- indications for escharotomy: decreased venous return, ventilatory compromise

(D) Because children have more compliant chest walls, circumferential thorax burns are particularly hazardous.

(E) BSAB > 15% are associated with paralytic ileus, leading to gastric distention.

(F) Monitor urine output closely. The most common cause of oliguria is inadequate fluid administration.

Increased fluid requirements are associated with inhalation and electrical injuries, fractures, edema formation, delayed resuscitation, and concomitant alcohol intoxication. See p. 144 for management of acute renal failure and treatment of myoglobinuria.

(G) **Morphine sulfate** 0.1-0.15 mg/kg IV (NOT IM/SC) **only after** adequate circulation is established and significant associated injuries are ruled out. If the patient does not respond to this measure, rule out other causes of agitation (occult trauma, early shock, hypoxia).

(H) Most injuries are associated with low voltage (<120 V) AC current (children biting plugs or extension cords). Electrical injuries are associated with myoglobinuria (See p 147). Maintain adequate hydration.

Smoke Inhalation Injury and Carbon Monoxide Poisoning

Mary Lieh-Lai and Michelle Rotta

> Smoke inhalation injury becomes evident in the airways, lungs and respiratory system within the first 5 days following the inhalation of thermal and chemical products of combustion.

(A) Chemical injury can occur at any level of the respiratory tract.

sulfur/nitrous oxides + lung H_2O	corrosive acids
burning wood ——————➤	CO
cotton/plastics combustion ——➤	aldehydes causing protein denaturation and cellular damage
polyvinylchloride ——————➤	chlorine and HCl released
polyethylene ——————————➤	hydrocarbons, ketones, and other acids
polyurethane ——————————➤	cyanide gas

(B) Thermal injury is usually limited to the upper airway (above the glottis).

Upper airway lesions are usually due to thermal inhalation injury including actual burns as well as severe edema of the naso/oropharynx and laryngeal structures. In severely hypovolemic patients, supraglottic edema may not manifest until after fluid resuscitation is initiated.

Lower airway lesions (below the glottis) are usually the results of chemical inhalation injury.

- Immediate effects of smoke inhalation include loss of ciliary action, mucosal edema, bronchiolitis, alveolar epithelial damage, and impaired gas exchange (oxygenation > ventilation). Areas of atelectasis worsen V/Q mismatch.
- Later effects: sloughing of tracheobronchial mucosa and mucopurulent membrane formation, increased likelihood of infection
- > 24 hr: Pathology similar to adult respiratory distress syndrome

(C) **Signs of respiratory distress can sometimes be delayed 12-24 hr, however they may be present from the start. Auscultatory findings precede chest radiographic abnormalities usually by 12-24 hr.**

(D) Radiographs may show diffuse interstitial infiltration or local areas of atelectasis and edema.

(E) CO poisoning is a significant cause of early death related to fires. It is also encountered with the use of improperly vented stoves, faulty or rear-vented exhaust systems in open trucks, faulty or unvented fireplaces, etc.

✳(Continued on p 192)

Clinical manifestations

History: Was the patient unconscious or was there neurologic impairment? Did the injury occur in a closed space? Were there noxious chemicals? Was CPR performed?

HEENT   facial burns, singed eyebrows or nasal hair, carbon deposits on mucosa, inflammatory changes of the oropharynx, carbonaceous sputum

RESP   hoarseness, grunting, tachypnea, wheezing, stridor

(D) **Diagnostics**

ABG/CBG with COHb level, cyanide level, chest radiograph

Suspected Inhalational Injury/ CO Poisoning

Stop the burning process	→ **Ensure ABCs. Stabilize C-spine.**
• remove all clothing. • copious irrigation of chemical burns (<u>min</u>. 20 min for chemical eye injuries) • remove all jewelry (rings, bracelets, watchbands).	→ 100% oxygen → **Burn management** (See p 186) Volume expansion in presence of cutaneous burns

← - -NOT indicated- - →

1. Steroids to reduce inflammation
2. Prophylactic antibiotics

UPPER AIRWAY INJURY	**LOWER AIRWAY INJURY**	☆**CO POISONING**
Obstruction can proceed very rapidly. Indications for intubation: • altered mental status • circumferential burns of lips, neck • intraoral burns of lips, neck • early (< 12 hr) occurrence of stridor, dyspnea, retractions Aggressive pulmonary toilet	Same as in upper airway injury Reflex bronchospasm secondary to chemical and particulate irritation of upper airway may contribute to lower airway obstruction. Consider trial of bronchodilators (**nebulized albuterol**).	Suspect in all fire victims and obtain COHb level. • ABG/CBG, CPR • **100% O₂** • pulse oximeter • treat metabolic acidosis with NaHCO₃ (See p 164). • consider cyanide poisoning if COHb > 20% with persistent metabolic acidosis.

☆ Hyperbaric O_2 has not been shown to be of more benefit than 100% O_2; in addition, it is not easily accessible. Do not delay resuscitation efforts in attempts to institute hyperbaric O_2 therapy.

✳(Continued from p 190)

(F) CO poisoning

COHb level	Manifestation
0.3-1.0% (endogenous)	None
1-10% (asymptomatic)	Increased threshold to visual stimuli, decreased angina threshold
20-40% (moderate toxicity)	Irritability, vomiting, tachycardia, shock
40-60% (severe toxicity)	Seizures, coma, vascular collapse
> 60%	Death

(G)   Classic red or pink color may be due to thermal injury. Patients may also be pale secondary to vasoconstriction.

(H) $t_{1/2}$ of COHb in room air is 4 hr. Half life is reduced to 1 hr when 100% oxygen is administered.

(I)   **Pulse oximeter readings are unreliable with COHb (See p 170).**

Notes

Trauma

Stabilization of the Trauma Patient

Michelle Rotta

> Trauma is defined in terms of extent (local vs. multiple), mechanism (blunt vs. penetrating) and severity. It is the **number one** cause of death in children > 1 yr of age in the US. 80% of all pediatric trauma is secondary to blunt injury. The most common causes of traumatic deaths in decreasing order are motor vehicular accidents (approximately 50%), homicide, suicide, drowning, pedestrian/motor vehicular accidents, and burns.

(A) The Pediatric GCS: 14-15 = normal and ≤ 8 represents severe neurologic deficit/injury. Patients with GCS ≤ 8 require intubation. CT scan of the head is recommended <u>only after</u> stabilization of airway and circulation.

The GCS and modification for children

Eye opening

4 Spontaneous
3 To speech
2 To pain
1 No response

Motor response

6 Spontaneous (obeys verbal commands)
5 Localizes pain
4 Withdraws to pain
3 Decorticate posture
2 Decerebrate posture
1 No response

Best verbal response

5 Oriented or	Social smile, orients to sound, follows objects, cooing, converses, interacts appropriately with environment
4 Confused/disoriented or	Consolable cries, aware of environment, uncooperative interactions
3 Inappropriate words or	Inappropriate persistent cries, moaning, inconsistently aware of environment/ inconsistenly consolable
2 Incomprehensible sounds or	Agitated, restless, inconsolable cries, unaware of environment
1 No Response	No response

From Rubenstein JS, Hageman JR. Monitoring of critically ill infants and children. *Crit Care Clin* 4:621, 1988.

*(Continued on p 196)

"Assume every injury exists until proven otherwise."

Multiple Trauma Victim

Primary survey/resuscitation

Airway management
C-spine stabilization

1. Provide 100% O_2. Monitoring:
   pulse oximeter, CR monitor
2. Maintain "sniffing position" using
   chin lift or jaw thrust.
3. Remove secretions, foreign body,
   or loose teeth.

☆ Oral intubation (See p 207) if
neurologic impairment is such that
the patient cannot protect airway
(Pediatric GCS ≤ 8) **(A)**

Notify General Surgery. ☎ _____

➤ Assume C-spine injury until
proven otherwise.

➤ Bag and mask ventilation almost
always provides effective
breathing.
  • Surgical and/or needle
    cricothyroidotomy is rarely
    indicated for the infant or
    small child.

Breathing

"Look, listen, feel."
Note patient's color, rate, and
pattern of breathing.

➤ • Assess vital signs **(B)**
    (appropriate for age)

Rule out tension pneumothorax,
massive hemothorax
decreased or unequal breath
sounds
unequal chest wall movement
tracheal deviation, crepitations
subcutaneous emphysema.
Thoracentesis (See p 219)

Auscultate under axillae to reduce
interference from transmitted
upper airway sounds.

➤ • Children can suffer internal
    injuries without external evi-
    dence secondary to compliant
    chest walls.
  • Consider early gastric decom-
    pression to allow full dia-
    phragmatic movement.
  • Insert <u>orogastric</u> tubes in
    patients with known or sus-
    pected facial trauma. ☆

Circulation

✳(Continued on p 197)

☆ Only the oral route should be used for both endotracheal
intubation and gastric tube insertion in cases of facial
injury and/or suspected basilar skull fracture.

Consider rapid sequence intubation (See p 212) in patients
with hemodynamic instability, orbital injury.

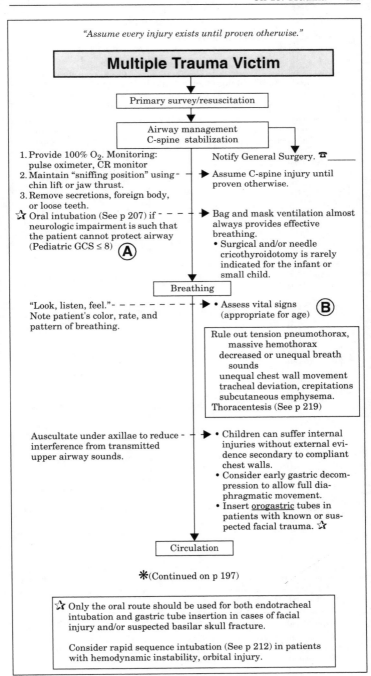

*(Continued from p 194)

Ⓑ **Table 15-1. Vital signs by age**

Age	Weight (kg)	Heart rate Range (beats/min)	Systolic blood pressure Range (mmHg)	Respiratory rate (breaths/min)
Preterm	2	120-180	40-60	55-65
Term newborn	3	90-170	52-92	40-60
1 month	4	110-180	60-104	30-50
6 month	7	110-180	65-125	25-35
1 yr	10	80-160	70-118	20-30
2 yr	12	80-130	73-117	20-30
4 yr	16	80-120	65-117	20-30
6 yr	20	75-115	76-116	18-24
8 yr	25	70-110	79-119	18-22
10 yr	30	70-110	82-122	16-20
12 yr	40	60-110	84-128	16-20
14 yr	50	60-105	84-136	16-20

From Iliff A, Lee VA. Pulse rate, respiratory rate, and body temperature of children between two months and eighteen years of age. *Child Dev* 23:237, 1952. With permission.

Table 15-2. The Pediatric Trauma Score.

PTS	+2	+1	-1
Airway	Normal	Oral/nasal airway	Intubated, tracheostomy invasive
Level of consciousness	Completely awake	Obtunded or any LOC	Comatose
Weight	> 20 kg	10-20 kg	< 10 kg
BP (systolic)	> 90 mmHg	50-90 mmHg	< 50 mmHg
Open wound	None	Minor	Major or penetrating
Fractures	None	Minor	Open or multiple fractures
Totals			

The Pediatric Trauma Score is used to assess injury severity, and is based on factors known to increase mortality and morbidity. A score of ≤ 8 indicates significant trauma, and these patients should be transferred to the nearest pediatric trauma center.

+2: pulse palpable at wrist; +1: pulse palpable at groin; -1: no pulse.

Adapted from the Committee on Trauma of the American College of Surgeons. *Advanced Trauma Life Support Course for Physicians.* 1989, p 265. American College of Surgeons. With permission.

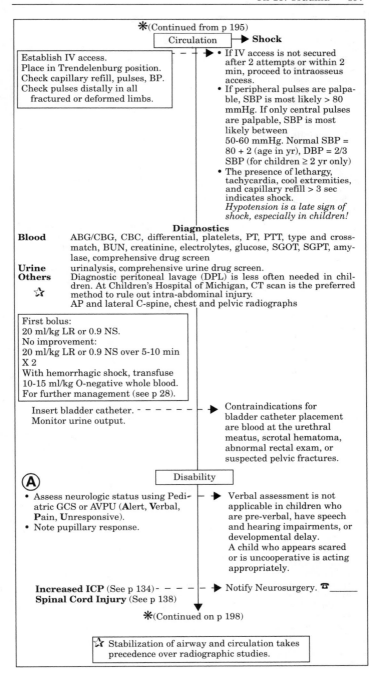

✳(Continued from p 195)

Circulation ──► **Shock**

Establish IV access.
Place in Trendelenburg position.
Check capillary refill, pulses, BP.
Check pulses distally in all
fractured or deformed limbs.

- If IV access is not secured after 2 attempts or within 2 min, proceed to intraosseus access.
- If peripheral pulses are palpable, SBP is most likely > 80 mmHg. If only central pulses are palpable, SBP is most likely between 50-60 mmHg. Normal SBP = 80 + 2 (age in yr), DBP = 2/3 SBP (for children ≥ 2 yr only)
- The presence of lethargy, tachycardia, cool extremities, and capillary refill > 3 sec indicates shock.
  Hypotension is a late sign of shock, especially in children!

Diagnostics

Blood ABG/CBG, CBC, differential, platelets, PT, PTT, type and cross-match, BUN, creatinine, electrolytes, glucose, SGOT, SGPT, amylase, comprehensive drug screen.

Urine urinalysis, comprehensive urine drug screen.

Others Diagnostic peritoneal lavage (DPL) is less often needed in children. At Children's Hospital of Michigan, CT scan is the preferred method to rule out intra-abdominal injury.
☆ AP and lateral C-spine, chest and pelvic radiographs

First bolus:
20 ml/kg LR or 0.9 NS.
No improvement:
20 ml/kg LR or 0.9 NS over 5-10 min
X 2
With hemorrhagic shock, transfuse
10-15 ml/kg O-negative whole blood.
For further management (see p 28).

Insert bladder catheter.
Monitor urine output.

──► Contraindications for bladder catheter placement are blood at the urethral meatus, scrotal hematoma, abnormal rectal exam, or suspected pelvic fractures.

Ⓐ   Disability

- Assess neurologic status using Pediatric GCS or AVPU (**A**lert, **V**erbal, **P**ain, **U**nresponsive).
- Note pupillary response.

──► Verbal assessment is not applicable in children who are pre-verbal, have speech and hearing impairments, or developmental delay.
A child who appears scared or is uncooperative is acting appropriately.

Increased ICP (See p 134) ──► Notify Neurosurgery. ☎_____
Spinal Cord Injury (See p 138)

✳(Continued on p 198)

☆ Stabilization of airway and circulation takes precedence over radiographic studies.

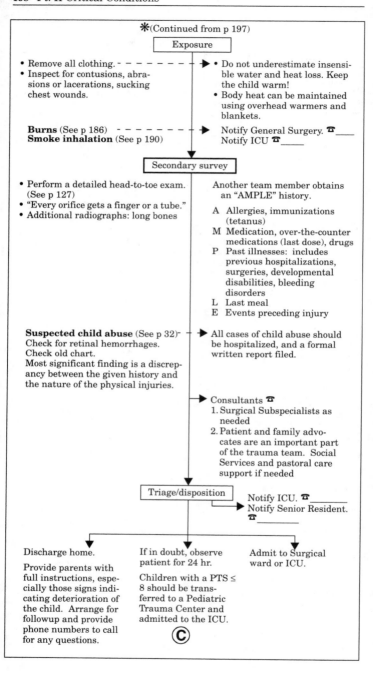

*(Continued from p 197)

Exposure

- Remove all clothing.
- Inspect for contusions, abrasions or lacerations, sucking chest wounds.

- Do not underestimate insensible water and heat loss. Keep the child warm!
- Body heat can be maintained using overhead warmers and blankets.

Burns (See p 186)
Smoke inhalation (See p 190)

Notify General Surgery. ☎____
Notify ICU ☎_____

Secondary survey

- Perform a detailed head-to-toe exam. (See p 127)
- "Every orifice gets a finger or a tube."
- Additional radiographs: long bones

Another team member obtains an "AMPLE" history.

A Allergies, immunizations (tetanus)
M Medication, over-the-counter medications (last dose), drugs
P Past illnesses: includes previous hospitalizations, surgeries, developmental disabilities, bleeding disorders
L Last meal
E Events preceding injury

Suspected child abuse (See p 32)
Check for retinal hemorrhages.
Check old chart.
Most significant finding is a discrepancy between the given history and the nature of the physical injuries.

All cases of child abuse should be hospitalized, and a formal written report filed.

Consultants ☎
1. Surgical Subspecialists as needed
2. Patient and family advocates are an important part of the trauma team. Social Services and pastoral care support if needed

Triage/disposition

Notify ICU. ☎_____
Notify Senior Resident. ☎_____

Discharge home.

Provide parents with full instructions, especially those signs indicating deterioration of the child. Arrange for followup and provide phone numbers to call for any questions.

If in doubt, observe patient for 24 hr.

Children with a PTS ≤ 8 should be transferred to a Pediatric Trauma Center and admitted to the ICU.

Admit to Surgical ward or ICU.

Ⓒ

Procedures

16 Commonly Performed Procedures in Pediatric Acute Care

- Abdominal Paracentesis
- Arterial Puncture
- Double Volume Exchange Transfusion
- Femoral Vein Cannulation
- Intraosseous Needle Placement
- Intubation
- Partial Exchange Transfusion
- Percutaneous Pericardiocentesis
- Rapid Sequence Intubation
- Subclavian Catheter Placement
- Subdural Tap
- Suprapubic Bladder Aspiration
- Thoracentesis: Needle Aspiration of Pneumothorax
- Umbilical Vein Cannulation

Commonly Performed Procedures in Pediatric Acute Care

Abdominal Paracentesis

Mary Lieh-Lai

> Indications: ascites - diagnostic or therapeutic

Equipment/supplies

- Documentation of amount of ascites with ultrasonography is helpful.
- sterile gloves, drapes
- 30- and 60-ml syringes
- 1% lidocaine
- tubes for sample collection (sterile)
- 4 x 4 gauze, Betadine solution
- 14-gauge or 16-gauge angiocatheter
- IV tubing
- 3-way stopcock

Procedure

1. Empty patient's bladder.
2. Elevate patient's head and chest to 30°. The patient may need sedation.
3. Clean abdominal area with Betadine.
4. Drape patient, using sterile technique.
5. Prepare 3-way stopcock with lever closed to middle port, connect one end to IV tubing, and connect tubing to 30 or 60 ml syringe.
6. Site: infraumbilical (see diagram)
7. Anesthetize site.
8. Using Z-track technique, insert the angiocatheter into the peritoneal cavity with continuous gentle aspiration on the syringe.
9. Remove needle and advance angiocatheter.
10. Aspirate as much peritoneal fluid as needed.
11. Send fluid for lab studies: RBC and WBC count with differential, amylase, Gram stain, protein, glucose, LDH, bacterial/viral/fungal cultures as indicated. If a malignancy is suspected, may need to notify Hematology/Oncology service, as well as Surgical Pathology for cell block studies.
12. Remove angiocatheter and apply dressing.
13. Procedure note

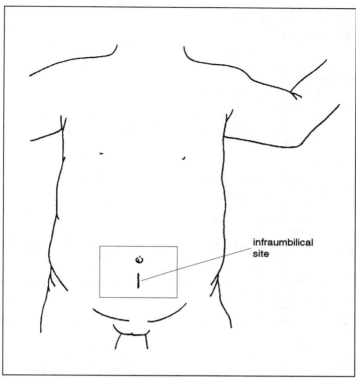

infraumbilical
site

Figure 16-1.   Abdominal paracentesis.

Arterial Puncture

Mary Lieh-Lai

> Indication: for arterial blood gases

Equpment/supplies

- 20-gauge butterfly needle
- alcohol and Betadine wipes
- tuberculin syringe with a minute amount of heparin (too much heparin can result in a falsely low pH)
- 2 x 2 or 4 x 4 gauze

Procedure

1. Refer to diagram for landmarks of radial artery.
2. Assure patency of ulnar collaterals with Allen test.
3. Clean area with Betadine and alcohol.
4. Attach tuberculin syringe to butterfly needle, unless using arterial blood sampler (e.g., Smooth-E).
5. With one finger on radial pulse, insert needle approximately 30° angle into the skin, aim toward pulse. Start aspirating when you see flashback.
6. After needle removal, apply steady pressure on area for at least 5 minutes.
7. Procedure note.

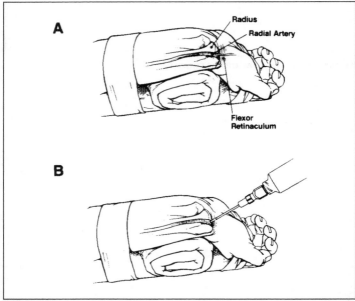

Figure 16-2. Arterial puncture. (From L Chameides, *Textbook of Pediatric Advanced Life Support*. Dallas: American Heart Association, 1994, p. 45. With permission.)

Double Volume Exchange Transfusion

Mary Lieh-Lai

Indications:	hyperbilirubinemia
	sepsis/DIC - e.g., meningococcemia
	acute leukemia with WBC > 250,000/mm^3

Equipment/supplies

- One central venous and one arterial line are preferred. If unavailable, 2 large-bore venous lines can be used, but this may make the procedure difficult, especially in larger patients.
- 4-way or 6-way stopcock.
- Tubing: one line connected to a container for discarded blood; one connected to a filter and transfusion bag
- 10-, 20-, or 60-ml syringes depending on aliquots planned
- Sterile drapes, gloves, gown
- Type and crossmatched PRBC reconstituted with FFP. (total volume: 160 ml/kg)
- If a large volume of blood is going to be used, it may be necessary to administer Ca^{+2} and glucose IV to the patient during the procedure.
- CR monitor
- Progress note or exchange transfusion sheet, and an assistant to record ins and outs.

Procedure

1. Obtain pre-exchange blood work: CBC, differential, total and direct bilirubin, PT, PTT, TT, Coomb's, serum electrolytes, glucose, Ca^{+2}, P.
2. Blood should be at room or near body temperature.
3. Have equipment ready. This procedure is preferably done with two individuals—one removing blood from the arterial catheter, and the other administering fresh blood into the venous line. Aliquots can be 5-ml, 10-ml, 20-ml, or 60-ml removed or administered depending on patient size.
4. Remember to administer Ca^{+2} and glucose as needed during the procedure.
5. Monitor vital signs, O_2 saturation.
6. Obtain post-exchange labs: same as pre-exchange labs.
7. Procedure note

Femoral Vein Cannulation

Jolene Ellis

Equipment/supplies
- 1% lidocaine
- vascular access tray
- syringes
- sterile drape
- 4 x 4 gauze, povidone-iodine solution
- suture kit

Procedure

1. Place patient on back with leg externally rotated (frog leg).
2. Palpate the femoral pulse. The femoral vein lies medially.
3. Prep and drape area using sterile technique.
4. Anesthetize the area with 1% lidocaine.
5. Insert needle medial to femoral pulse 1-2 cm below inguinal ligament.
6. Advance needle at 45° angle directed at umbilicus until free flow of blood is obtained.
7. After successful cannulation of vessel, complete procedure using the Seldinger technique.
8. Check and secure placement of CVC by radiograph.
9. Procedure note

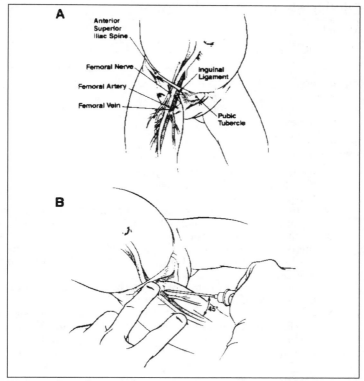

Figure 16-3.   Femoral vein cannulation. (From L Chameides, *Textbook of Pediatric Advanced Life Support.* **Dallas:American Heart Association, 1994, p. 42. With permission.)**

Intraosseous Needle Placement

Mary Lieh-Lai

> Indication: for vascular access when venous route cannot be established.

Equipment/supplies
- IO needles, hemostat
- IV tubing, IV solution
- Betadine
- 4 x 4 gauze

Procedure

1. Preferred site in children: upper tibia
2. See illustration for landmarks.
3. Cleanse area thoroughly with Betadine.
4. Hold IO needle between index and middle finger and thumb. Insert the needle at a right angle to the tibia, but aiming towards the foot. With slow and gentle rocking/twisting motion, enter IO space. Unscrew "door-knob-like" attachment from needle. Attach IV tubing to needle.
5. Clamp needle with hemostat at the level of the skin, and secure to limb.

Note: blood return is not always evident, even with successful entry, but always ascertain placement. Needle placement in SC or muscle tissue leads to undesired complications.

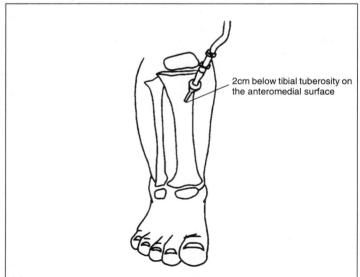

2cm below tibial tuberosity on the anteromedial surface

Figure 16-4.   Introsseous needle placement.

Intubation

Joan Less

> Indications (partial list): respiratory failure, upper airway obstruction, neuromuscular weakness with respiratory failure, hemodynamic instability, emergent drug administration, hyperventilation for increased ICP.

Equipment/supplies

- bag and appropriate size mask with O_2 source, reservoir
- laryngoscope handle
- laryngoscope blade with light bulb
- endotracheal tube
- wall suction
- suction catheter or Yankauer suction device
- gloves
- tincture of benzoin compound
- tape
- stylet (optional)
- Magill forceps for nasotracheal intubation only
- lubricant, for nasotracheal intubation only
- pulse oximeter, EKG monitor
- phenylephrine 0.25% solution for nasotracheal intubation only

Procedure

Orotracheal intubation

1. Provide 100% O_2 via bag and mask ventilation.
2. Have all equipment ready and available.
3. Attach pulse oximeter probe and EKG monitor to patient.
4. Sedate and paralyze patient with appropriate agents.
5. Ascertain integrity of spinal column.
6. Place patient supine in "sniffing" position. Slightly extend neck; use neck roll if extra support desired (contraindicated in spinal cord injury).
7. Attach laryngoscope blade to laryngoscope handle; ascertain that light bulb is securely in place and in working condition.
8. Place laryngoscope blade in right corner of mouth.
9. Direct laryngoscope to the left and into the pharynx, displacing the tongue.
10. Hold handle at 45°.
11. Lift handle to displace mandible and visualize the vocal cords; avoid pressure on the gums, teeth, and lips while displacing the mandible.
12. Slight pressure on the cricoid region may be required to visualize the cords (Sellick maneuver).
13. Suction oral secretions if necessary.
14. Advance endotracheal tube from the right corner of the mouth into the larynx; do not direct the endotracheal tube through the laryngoscope blade.

15. While holding the endotracheal tube in place, attach bag and provide manual ventilation with 100% O_2.
16. Moisture condensation in the endotracheal tube indicates that the tube is most likely in the trachea.
17. Check for equal and bilateral breath sounds and chest excursion while providing manual ventilation.
18. During intubation, another observer should monitor pulse oximeter and EKG readings.
19. Apply tincture of benzoin compound to perioral area, and tape tube securely in place.
20. Obtain STAT chest radiograph to assess whether the tip of the endotracheal tube is at the correct position.
21. Procedure note

Nasotracheal intubation (contraindicated in coagulopathy, basilar skull fractures, and severe injuries to the hypopharynx)
1. Provide 100% O_2 via bag and mask ventilation.
2. Have all equipment ready and available.
3. Attach pulse oximeter probe and EKG monitor to patient.
4. Sedate and paralyze the patient with appropriate agents.
5. Ascertain integrity of spinal column.
6. Place patient supine in "sniffing" position. Slightly extend neck; use neck roll if extra support desired (contraindicated in spinal cord injury).
7. Apply topical vasoconstrictor (such as phenylephrine 0.25%) to nasal mucosa.
8. Guide lubricated endotracheal tube into the nasal cavity; direct endotracheal tube posteriorly so that it enters the nasopharynx.
9. Visualize nasal tube tip in the nasopharynx.
10. Advance endotracheal tube to vocal cords. Magill forceps may be used to advance tube.
11. Advance endotracheal tube past vocal cords.
12. Moisture condensation in the endotracheal tube indicates that the tube is most likely in the trachea.
13. Check for equal and bilateral breath sounds and chest excursion while providing manual ventilation.
14. During intubation, another observer should monitor pulse oximeter and EKG readings.
15. Apply tincture of benzoin compound to nasal area and tape tube securely in place.
16. Obtain STAT chest radiograph to assess whether the tip of the endotracheal tube is at the correct position.
17. Procedure note

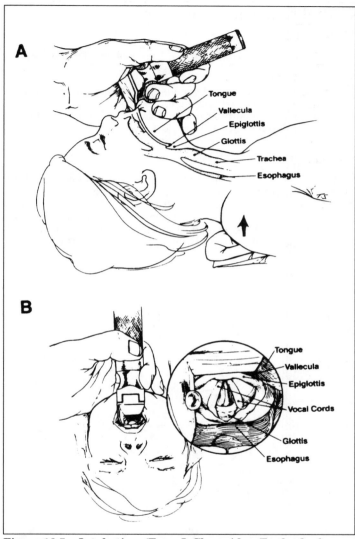

Figure 16-5.   Intubation. (From L Chameides, *Textbook of Pediatric Advanced Life Support*. Dallas:American Heart Association, 1994, p. 30. With permission.)

Partial Exchange Transfusion

Mary Lieh-Lai

> Indication: in sickle cell crisis, to reduce the amount of sickled cells

Equipment/supplies

- peripheral or central venous line. Peripheral catheter should be at least 20 gauge.
- sufficient amount of properly typed and crossmatched packed red cells (10-12 ml/kg)
- container for discarded blood

Procedure

1. After starting and securing IV access, remove 5 ml/kg of patient's blood. Monitor vital signs closely.
2. Transfuse 10-12 ml/kg PRBC.
3. If the patient is hemodynamically unstable, remove only 2 ml/kg, transfuse 5 ml/kg PRBC; remove additional 3 ml/kg, then transfuse 5-7 ml/kg PRBC.
4. Procedure note.

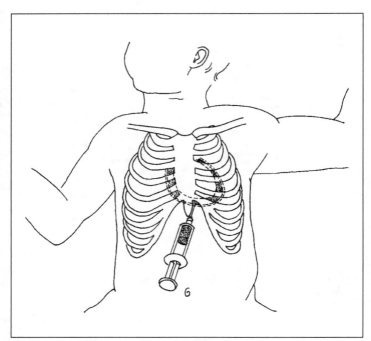

Figure 16-6.   Percutaneous pericardiocentesis.

Percutaneous Pericardiocentesis

Mary Lieh-Lai

> Indication: pericardial tamponade (air or fluid). Confirm diagnosis by radiograph and echocardiogram.

Equipment/supplies
- 4 x 4 gauze
- Betadine solution
- sterile gloves, gown
- sterile drapes
- 1% lidocaine
- 14- or 16-gauge angiocatheter
- 10- and 60-ml syringes
- 3-way stopcock
- specimen tubes (if fluid is being collected)
- sedative medications
- CR monitor
- pulse oximeter
- code cart
- plasmanate or other volume expanders at the bedside
- alligator clamp (if available) attached to EKG monitor

Procedure

1. Sedate patient if necessary.
2. Anesthetize area with lidocaine.
3. See illustration for landmarks.
4. Use sterile technique.
5. Patient can be supine or sitting upright at 45° angle.
6. Set up 3-way stopcock with lever off to middle port. Attach syringe to stopcock.
7. Attach alligator clamp to hub of angiocatheter.
8. Insert angiocatheter under the left subxiphoid region and direct it toward the patient's left shoulder at approximately 45° while continuously aspirating. As the pericardial space is entered, a "popping" sensation will be felt, followed by free aspiration of fluid or air. With alligator clamp in place, the EKG monitor will show an extra "spike" indicating pericardial injury (and entry). Remove needle and quickly place thumb to cover the angiocath opening. Attach 3-way stopcock with syringe and start aspirating. Collect fluid into specimen tubes as necessary.
9. Send fluid for labs: bacterial/viral/fungal cultures, cell count, differential, glucose, protein, LDH, Gram stain, amylase.
10. During the procedure, monitor patient carefully; watch for dysrhythmias.
11. Remove needle and apply dressing.
12. Repeat chest radiograph and echocardiogram.
13. Continue to monitor patient every 15 min for the next few hours.
14. Procedure note

Rapid Sequence Intubation

Katherine Ling-McGeorge

> Indications: to maintain adequate oxygenation, protect the airway, reduce adverse cardiovascular responses to intubation

Succinylcholine and other neuromuscular blocking agents should only be used by physicians who understand their pharmacologic actions, who are familiar with procedures to secure the airway, and have appropriate medical assistance to carry out these procedures, along with the availability of monitoring equipment.

(A) Nondepolarizing agents such as vecuronium and atracurium reduce fasciculations associated with the use of succinylcholine, thereby eliminating the risk of increasing intracranial, intraocular, and gastric pressures during the procedure.

Reversal: **neostigmine** 2.5 mg and **glycopyrrolate** (Robinol) 0.5 mg in a single syringe, slow IV push. Glycopyrrolate is used to counter the cholinergic effects of neostigmine.

(B) Atracurium spontaneously dissociates into inert by-products by a process known as Hoffman elimination. It is preferred in patients with liver or renal impairment, because its metabolism is independent of hepatic or renal function.

(C) Atropine reduces the incidence of bradycardia.

(D) Lidocaine reduces vagal response to intubation.

(E) Midazolam is a short-acting benzodiazepine with additional amnestic properties. May be associated with respiratory depression when administered IV.

Reversal: **flumazenil** 0.2 mg IV over 30 sec, repeat after 30 sec using 0.3 mg, then 0.5 mg for further dosing, <u>max</u>. 5 mg. Seizures may be induced with the use of flumazenil in the following cases: patients with concomitant cyclic antidepressant ingestion, patients addicted to benzodiazepines.

(F) The use of fentanyl has been associated with chest wall rigidity in some patients.

Reversal: **naloxone** 0.1 mg/kg IV.

(G) Morphine sulfate and thiopental may be associated with hypotension resulting from vasodilatory effects.

Avoid thiopental in patients with hypotension or status asthmaticus.

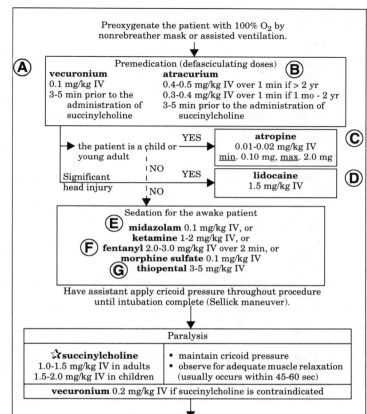

Preoxygenate the patient with 100% O_2 by nonrebreather mask or assisted ventilation.

(A)   Premedication (defasciculating doses)   (B)

vecuronium	**atracurium**
0.1 mg/kg IV	0.4-0.5 mg/kg IV over 1 min if > 2 yr
3-5 min prior to the	0.3-0.4 mg/kg IV over 1 min if 1 mo - 2 yr
administration of	3-5 min prior to the administration of
succinylcholine	succinylcholine

the patient is a child or → YES → **atropine** (C)
young adult | 0.01-0.02 mg/kg IV
      |NO   <u>min</u>. 0.10 mg, <u>max</u>. 2.0 mg

Significant → YES → **lidocaine** (D)
head injury |NO   1.5 mg/kg IV

Sedation for the awake patient
(E)   **midazolam** 0.1 mg/kg IV, or
    ketamine 1-2 mg/kg IV, or
(F) **fentanyl** 2.0-3.0 mg/kg IV over 2 min, or
   morphine sulfate 0.1 mg/kg IV
   (G)   **thiopental** 3-5 mg/kg IV

Have assistant apply cricoid pressure throughout procedure until intubation complete (Sellick maneuver).

Paralysis	
☆**succinylcholine**	• maintain cricoid pressure
1.0-1.5 mg/kg IV in adults	• observe for adequate muscle relaxation
1.5-2.0 mg/kg IV in children	(usually occurs within 45-60 sec)
vecuronium 0.2 mg/kg IV if succinylcholine is contraindicated	

Oral intubation
• If unable to secure airway within 20-30 seconds, stop procedure and ventilate patient with bag and mask and 100% O_2 for 1-2 minutes before reattempting to intubate.
• If paralysis is inadequate, repeat dose of succinylcholine at 1.0-1.5 mg/kg IV. ☆

Verify placement by auscultation; ensure equality of breath sounds.
Secure endotracheal tube.
Verify position with chest radiograph.

☆ Contraindications to succinylcholine: crush injuries, burns, increased ICP, hyperkalemia, neuromuscular disorders, pseudocholinesterase deficiency, malignant hyperthermia, orbital injuries

Subclavian Catheter Placement

Jolene Ellis

Equipment/supplies

- lidocaine 1%
- vascular access tray
- syringes
- sterile drapes, gloves, gown
- 4 x 4 gauze, povidone-iodine solution
- suture kit

Procedure

1. Place child in Trendelenburg position with head turned away from side desired for venous access.
2. Identify suprasternal notch, middle and medial third of clavicle, and pectoral shoulder groove. See illustration for landmark.
3. Prep and drape area using sterile technique.
4. Anesthetize the area with 1% lidocaine.
5. Introduce the needle at the junction of the middle and medial third of the clavicle directed toward the index finger placed on the suprasternal notch.
6. The syringe should be parallel to the frontal plane.
7. Apply negative pressure to the syringe and advance needle under the clavicle toward the suprasternal notch.
8. When free flow of blood is achieved, rotate bevel downward 90° to encourage placement of the catheter into the superior vena cava. Place thumb over the needle hub when disconnecting syringe to prevent air entry/ embolism.
9. Complete the procedure using Seldinger technique.
10. Check catheter placement by radiograph.
11. Procedure note

Note: subclavian venous access has a high rate of complications in infants and young children (such as pneumothorax) when performed emergently, therefore, other routes are preferable.

See Figure 16-7 on page 215.

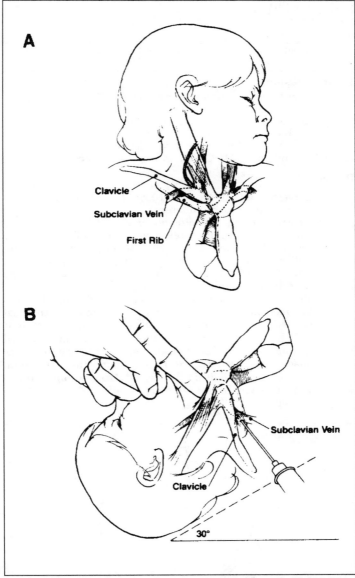

Figure 16-7.   Subclavian vein cannulation. (From L Chameides, *Textbook of Pediatric Advanced Life Support.* **Dallas: American Heart Association, 1994, p. 43. With permission.)**

Subdural Tap

Mary Lieh-Lai

> Indications: emergent evacuation of subdural fluid to relieve
> increased ICP

Equipment/supplies
- 19- or 20-gauge subdural or spinal needle (check patency first)
- 10-ml syringe
- shaving kit
- Betadine and 70% alcohol, sterile gauze
- bag and mask, O_2, CR monitor, pulse oximeter

Procedure
1. Have bag and mask with 100% O_2 available as well as CR monitor, pulse oximeter.
2. Restrain infant in supine position.
3. Shave scalp around lateral boundaries of the anterior fontanelle. Cleanse area with Betadine and 70% alcohol; dry with sterile gauze. Wearing sterile gloves, palpate the coronal suture at the lateral aspect of the anterior fontanelle.
4. Firmly grasp subdural or spinal needle by the hub between the thumb and index finger, and rest the heel of the hand against the infant's scalp. Puncture skin at 90° angle using Z-track technique. Advance needle until a "pop" is felt. This indicates entry into the subdural space. Do not advance needle more than 5-8 mm. Remove stylet to drain fluid/blood. **Do not aspirate.**
5. Replace stylet before removing needle.
6. Procedure note.

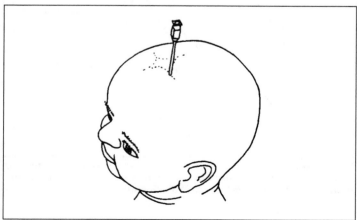

Figure 16-8.   Subdural tap.

Suprapubic Bladder Aspiration

Mary Lieh-Lai

> Indication: when sterile urine culture is necessary. Avoid in patients with genitourinary tract anomalies.

Equipment/supplies
- Betadine and 70% alcohol
- 22- or 24-gauge 1-inch needle
- 10-ml syringe

Procedure

1. Ascertain that the infant has not voided in the past 60 min before the procedure.
2. Restrain the infant in the frog-leg position.
3. Clean suprapubic area (see diagram) with Betadine and 70% alcohol.
4. With needle attached to the syringe, enter the bladder 2 cm above the symphysis pubis in the midline. Aim caudally. Apply gentle suction to the syringe until urine is obtained. Do not advance needle more than 2.5 cm.
5. Remove needle.
6. Procedure note

See Figure 16-9 on page 218.

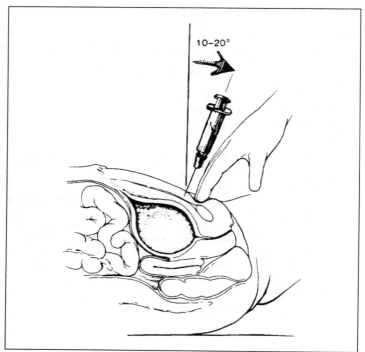

Figure 16-9. Suprapubic bladder aspiration. (From GR Fleisher and S Ludwig (eds), *Textbook of Pediatric Emergency Medicine*. Baltimore: Williams and Wilkins, 1993, p. 1646. with permission.)

Thoracentesis:
Needle Aspiration of Pneumothorax

Mary Lieh-Lai

> Indication: pneumothorax with cardiovascular compromise

Equipment/supplies

- 20-gauge or 18-gauge angiocatheter
- 3-way stopcock
- 60-ml syringe
- Betadine, 4 x 4 gauze
- sterile drapes
- sterile gloves, masks
- CR monitor
- pulse oximeter
- petrolatum-impregnated gauze

Procedure

1. Cleanse area with Betadine.
2. Prep and drape area, using sterile technique.
3. With patient supine, locate the 2nd intercostal space at the midclavicular line on the side with the pneumothorax. Make sure the 3-way stopcock lever is turned such that it is off to the middle port. Attach syringe to the stopcock. With a syringe attached to the angiocatheter, approach the area at about a 45° angle. Enter the pleural cavity between the ribs, staying close to the superior border of the rib to avoid hitting blood vessels and nerves. Continue aspirating while advancing the needle. A popping sensation is usually felt when the intrapleural space is entered. Remove needle, attach the stopcock with syringe attached to the angiocatheter and aspirate. To "discard" aspirated air, turn stopcock lever off to patient and discard through middle port. Continue to aspirate intrapleural air in this fashion, until you can no longer get air without meeting resistance.
4. Apply petrolatum occlusive dressing to area after catheter removal.
5. Obtain post-thoracentesis radiograph.
6. Procedure note
   See Figure 16-10 on page 220.

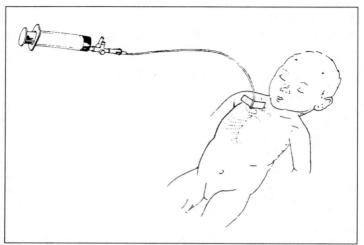

Figure 16-10.   Thoracentesis: needle aspiration of pneumothorax. (From HL Halliday, G McCluire, and H Reid (eds), *Handbook of Neonatal Intensive Care.* **Philadelphia: WB Saunders Co., 1989, p. 93. With permission.)**

Umbilical Vein Cannulation

Jolene Ellis

Equipment/supplies
- 3.5 or 5.0 Fr. single lumen catheter
- sterile measuring tape, umbilical tape
- sterile drapes, gloves, gown
- 3 way stopcock
- syringe with saline flush, povidone-iodine solution
- 4 x 4 gauze
- scalpel, blade, needle holder, sutures
- dilator

Procedure

1. Secure infant in supine position.
2. Determine length of catheter to be inserted for either-high (T6-T9) or low (L3-L4) placement (See chart below).
3. Flush catheter with sterile saline solution before insertion.
4. Cleanse umbilical stump using sterile technique.
5. Tie umbilical string around base of umbilical stump.
6. Hold umbilical stump with hemostat and cut cord with a scalpel 2 cm above the skin line.
7. Normally, the umbilical vein is the thin-walled, single vessel that is larger than the two thicker-walled arteries. Gently dilate vessel.
8. Insert umbilical catheter into umbilical vein to desired length. Check for good blood return.
9. Secure catheter with suture and tape bridge.
10. Confirm placement of catheter by radiograph.

See Figures 16-11 and 16-12 on page 222.

11. Procedure note

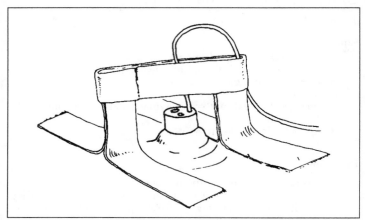

Figure 16-11. Umbilical vein cannulation and taping. (From HL Halliday, G McClure, and H Reid (eds), *Handbook of Neonatal Intensive Care*. Phiadelphia: WB Saunders Co., 1989, p. 99. With permission.)

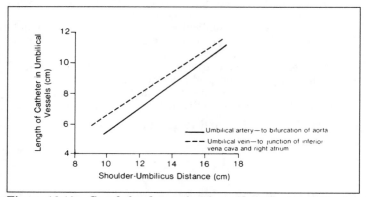

Figure 16-12. Graph for determination of length of umbilical catheter to be inserted. (From MA Fletcher and MG Macdonald (eds), Atlas of Procedures in Neonatology. Philadelphia: JB Lippincott Co., 1993, p. 156. With permission.)

Appendix

Antimicrobial Formulary Agents

**Table A-1. Antimicrobial Formulary Agents
Recommended Pediatric Doses**

Agent	Route	Dosage mg/kg/day	Interval	Max/ 24 hr	Comments
Acyclovir	IV	30	q 8 hr		Infuse over 1 hr.
Acyclovir	PO	80	QID	3.2 g	Give during day hours. Not for serious infections
Amikacin	IV, IM	15	q 8 hr	1.5 g	Obtain serum levels.
Amoxicillin	PO	25-50	q 6-8 hr	2 g	
Amoxicillin/ clavulanate (Augmentin)	PO	25-40	q 6-8 hr	1.5 g	Dose reflects amoxicillin component.
Amphotericin B	IV	1.0	q 24 hr		Start with 0.25 mg/kg dose. Protect from direct sunlight. Infuse over 6 hr.
Ampicillin	IV, IM	400 100-200	q 4 hr q 4 hr	12 g 12 g	Meningitis only All other infections
Ampicillin/ sulbactam (Unasyn)	IV, IM	100-200	q 4 hr	8 g	Dose reflects ampicillin component. Approved for ≥ 12 years
Cefazolin	IV, IM	50-100	q 8 hr	6 g	
Cefixime	PO	8	q 12-24 hr	400 mg	
Cefotaxime	IV, IM	160	q 6 hr	12 g	
Cefpodoxime	PO	10	q 12 hr	200 mg	
Ceftazidime	IV, IM	150	q 8 hr	6 g	
Ceftriaxone	IV, IM	50-100	q 12 hr	4 g	May cause jaundice and cholelithiasis.
Cefuroxime	IV, IM	150	q 8 hr	6 g	
Cefuroxime axetil (Ceftin)	PO	30	q 12 hr	2 g	
Cephalexin	PO	25-50	q 6 hr	4 g	
Chloramphenicol palmitate	PO	75	q 6 hr	3 g	Obtain serum levels.
Chloramphenicol succinate	IV	75-100	q 6 hr	3 g	
Clindamycin	IV	25-50	q 6-8 hr	4 g	
Clindamycin	PO	20-30	q 6 hr	2 g	
Cloxacillin	PO	50-100	q 6 hr	4 g	Check pharmacy for availability.
Dicloxacillin	PO	25-50	q 6 hr	2 g	Check pharmacy for availability.
Doxycycline	IV, PO	2-4	q 12 hr	200 mg	Patients > 8 yr
Erythromycin ethylsuccinate	PO	40-50	q 6 hr	2 g	

**Table A-1.   Antimicrobial Formulary Agents
Recommended Pediatric Doses (Continued)**

Agent	Route	Dosage mg/kg/day	Interval	Max/ 24 hr	Comments
EES/ sulfisoxazole (Pediazole)	PO	40-50	q 6 hr	2 g	Dose based on EES component
Erythromycin lactobionate	IV	20-40	q 6 hr	2 g	Infuse over 1-2 hr.
Gentamicin	IM, IV	5.0-7.5	q 8 hr	300 mg	Obtain serum levels.
Isoniazid	PO	10-20	q 12-24 hr	300 mg	
Ketoconazole	PO	5-10	q 12-24 hr	400 mg	
Methicillin	IV	200-400	q 4 hr	12 g	
Metronidazole	IV	30	q 6 hr	4 g	
Metronidazole	PO	15-35	q 8 hr	4 g	
Oxacillin	IV	100-200	q 4 hr	12 g	
Penicillin Benzathine Penicillin V Procaine Aqueous	IM <u>only</u> PO IM <u>only</u> IV, IM	50,000 U 25-50 50,000 U up to 400,000 U	1 dose q 6-8 hr q 12-24 hr q 4 hr	4.8 M U 3 g 4.8 M U 20 M U	
Piperacillin	IV	300	q 4 hr	20 g	
Ribavirin	inhaled	6-g vial	q 24 hr		3-5 days
Rifampin	PO PO PO	10-20 20 20	q 12-13 hr once/day q12 hr	600 mg 600 mg 600 mg	For TB 4 days for *Hemophilus influenza* prophylaxis 2 days for meningococcal pro- phylaxis
Ticarcillin	IV	200-400	q 4 hr	18 g	
Tobramycin	IM, IV	5.0-7.5	q 8 hr	300 mg	Obtain serum levels.
Trimethoprim- sulfamethox- azole (TMP/SMZ)	PO, IV PO, IV	8 TMP/ 40 SMZ 20 TMP/ 100 SMZ	q 8-12 hr q 6 hr	320 mg TMP 1.2 g TMP	For general infections For *Pneumocystis carinii* only
Vancomycin	PO IV	25-40 40	q 6 hr q 6 hr	2 g 2 g	For *Clostridium difficile* only Infuse over 1 hr. Obtain serum levels.

Samples of
Continuous Infusion Calculations

Dopamine for a child in cardiogenic shock

       weight   5 kg

       desired dose   10 µg/kg/minute

a)   Concentration is 200 µg of dopamine in 250 ml of D_5W

$$\frac{200mg}{250ml} = \frac{0.8mg}{ml} \times \frac{1000µg}{mg} = \frac{800µg}{ml}$$

$$\frac{800\ µg/ml}{5\ kg} \times \frac{10\ µg/kg/minute}{X\ ml}$$

$$800\ X = 50$$

$$X = \frac{50}{800} = 0.06\ ml/minute \times 60 = 3.75\ ml/hour\ (infusion\ rate)$$

b)   Concentration is 400 mg in 250 ml D_5W

$$\frac{400mg}{250ml} = \frac{1.6mg}{ml} \times \frac{1000µg}{mg} = \frac{1600µg}{ml}$$

$$\frac{1600\ µg/ml}{5\ kg} \times \frac{10\ µg/kg/minute}{X\ ml}$$

$$1600\ X = 50$$

$$X = \frac{50}{1600} = 0.03\ ml/minute \times 60 = 1.8\ ml/hour\ (infusion\ rate)$$

Isoproterenol for a child in status asthmaticus

       weight   20 kg

       desired dose   0.15 µg/kg/min

Concentration is 2 mg in 100 ml D_5W

$$\frac{2mg}{100ml} = \frac{0.02mg}{ml} \times \frac{1000µg}{mg} = \frac{20µg}{ml}$$

$$\frac{20\ µg/ml}{20\ kg} \times \frac{0.15\ µg/kg/minute}{X\ ml}$$

$$20\ X = 3$$

$$X = \frac{3}{20} = 0.15\ ml/minute \times 60 = 9\ ml/hour\ (infusion\ rate)$$

NOTE: Inotropic solutions generally come in standard mixtures. It is for this reason that the above calculations are more practical than the recommended formula,

$$6 \times \frac{desired\ dose(µg/kg/minute)}{desired\ rate\ (ml/hr)} \times wt\ (kg) = \frac{mg\ drug}{100\ ml\ of\ fluid}$$

where varying concentrations will be requested that may not always be available.

Formulae

Plasma osmolality	$\text{plasma osmolality} = 2(\text{Na}) + \dfrac{\text{glucose}}{18} + \dfrac{\text{BUN}}{2.8}$
Osmolar gap	$\text{osmolar gap} = (\text{measured osmolality} - \text{calculated osmolality})$
Anion gap	$\text{anion gap} = (\text{serum Na} + \text{K}) - (\text{Cl}^- + \text{HCO}_3^-)$
Alveolar O_2 pressure	$PAO_2 = \left[FIO_2 \times (PB - 47) \right] - \dfrac{PaCO_2}{R}$
A-a gradient	$AaDO_2 = PAO_2 - PaO_2$
Shunt fraction	$\dfrac{Qs}{Qt} = \dfrac{CcO_2 - CaO_2}{CcO_2 - C\bar{v}O_2}$
Arterial O_2 content	$CaO_2 = [\text{Hgb} \times 1.34 \times SaO_2] + [PaO_2 \times 0.003]$
Mixed venous O_2 content	$C\bar{v}O_2 = [\text{Hgb} \times 1.34 \times S\bar{v}O_2] + [P\bar{v}O_2 \times 0.003]$
Pulmonary end capillary O_2 content	$CcO_2 = [\text{Hgb} \times 1.34] + [PAO_2 \times 0.003]$
O_2 consumption	$VO_2 = [AVO_2 \times 10] \times \text{cardiac output}$
AV O_2 difference	$A\text{-}\bar{v}DO_2 = CaO_2 - C\bar{v}O_2$
Cardiac index	$CI = \dfrac{\text{Cardiac Output}}{\text{BSA}}$
Mean arterial pressure	$MAP = \dfrac{\text{systolic} + 2\,(\text{diastolic})}{3}$
Systemic vascular resistance	$SVR = \dfrac{80(\text{MAP-CVP})}{CI}$
Pulmonary vascular resistance	$PVR = \dfrac{80(\text{MPAP} - \text{PCWP})}{CI}$
Creatinine clearance	$CICr = \dfrac{(140 - \text{age})(\text{weight in kg})}{72 \times \text{serum Cr}}$
Renal failure index	$RFI = \dfrac{\text{Urine Na} \times \text{Serum Cr}}{\text{Urine Cr}}$
Fractional excretion of sodium	$FENa = \dfrac{\text{Urine Na} \times \text{Serum Cr}}{\text{Serum Na} \times \text{Urine Cr}} \times 100$
Centigrade	$^{\circ}C = (^{\circ}F - 32) \times 5/9$
Fahrenheit	$^{\circ}F = (^{\circ}C \times 9/5) + 32$
Size of ET tube	$\dfrac{\text{Age}}{4} + 4$

Table of Forced Vital Capacity Normalized for Weight and Height Values

Table D-1. Forced vital capacity values

Summary of Normal Values and SD* for Lung Volumes in Children

HEIGHT (cm.)	VC (ml.) Male Mean	±2SD	VC (ml.) Female Mean	±2SD	FEV₁.₀ (ml.) Male+Female Mean	±2SD	FRC (ml.) Male Mean	±2SD	FRC (ml.) Female Mean	±2SD	RV (ml.) Male Mean	±2SD	RV (ml.) Female Mean	±2SD	TLC (ml.) Male Mean	±2SD	TLC (ml.) Female Mean	±2SD
110	1252	216	1223	294	1053	258	662	356	693	244	369	130	369	130	1539	504	1513	496
120	1592	214	1554	260	1403	252	873	300	893	210	453	134	453	134	1980	374	1953	368
130	1979	230	1916	268	1457	228	1110	266	1118	204	545	130	545	130	2470	282	2437	242
140	2411	288	2323	300	2146	304	1375	270	1367	224	653	122	653	122	3016	270	2974	242
150	2883	400	2770	366	2586	412	1673	284	1643	266	773	118	773	118	3633	304	3576	326
160	3421	546	3270	502	3080	568	2003	318	1942	322	907	134	907	134	4308	444	4242	520
170	4038	802	3856	782	3629	724	2372	424	2323	452	1056	182	1056	182	5070	732	5039	822

*SD calculated for mean values by different authors around the overall mean.

From G Polgar and V Promadhat, *Pulmonary Function Testing in Children: Techniques and Standards*, Philadelphia: WB Saunders Co, p 255. With permission

ICU Card

Children's Hospital of Michigan
Division of Critical Care
A. Sarnaik, M. Lieh-Lai, K. Meert
(313) 745-0102

Table E-1. ICU card

Age	Internal diameter (mm)	Oral: mouth to midtrachea (cms)	Nasal: nare to midtrachea (cms)
Premature	2.5-3.0	9	10
Full-term	3.0-3.5	10	11
6 mos	4.0	11	13
12-24 mos	4.5	13-14	16-17
4 yr	5.0	15	17-18
6 yr	5.5	17	19-20
8 yr	6.0	19	21-22
10 yr	6.5	20	22-23
12 yr	7.0	21	23-24
14 yr	7.5	22	24-25
Adults	8-9.5	23-25	25-28

Table E-2. GCS

Eyes		
Open	Spontaneously	4
	To verbal command	3
	To pain	2
	No response	1
Best verbal		
	Oriented and conversant	5
	Disoriented and conversant	4
	Inappropriate words	3
	Incomprehensible sounds	2
	No response	1
Best motor		
To verbal command	Obeys	6
To painful stimulus	Localizes	5
	Flexion-withdrawal	4
	Flexion-abnormal (decorticate rigidity)	3
	Extension (decerebrate rigidity)	2
	No response	1
	Total	3-15

Table E-3. Therapeutic serum drug levels

Drug		Level
Carbamazepine		4-12 µg/ml
Clonazepam		15-70 µg/ml
Cyanide		< 0.5 mg/L
Cyclosporine (whole blood) early post-tx	trough	250-800 ng/ml (RIA) 100-450 ng/ml (HPLC)
Digoxin		0.8-2 ng/ml
Gentamicin/ tobramycin	peak trough	6-10 µg/ml <2 µg/ml
Lidocaine		2-6 µg/ml
Phenytoin		10-20 µg/ml
Theophylline (bronchospasm)		8-15 µg/ml
Thiocyanate		< 10 mg/dL
Valproic acid		50–150 µg/ml
Vancomycin	peak trough	30-40 µg/ml <7.5 µg/ml

Table E-4. Commonly used emergency drugs

Agent	Route	Dose	Frequency
Adenosine	IV	0.05-0.25 mg/kg	Increase by 0.05 mg/kg q 2 min up to 0.25 mg/kg
Atracurium	IV	0.4 mg/kg	q 1 hour
Atropine	IV	0.02 mg/kg minimum: 0.1 mg	once, repeat in 20 minutes
Bicarbonate	IV	1 mEq/kg over 15 to 30 min	
Bretylium	IV	5 mg/kg	q 1-2 hr
Bumetanide	IV, PO	0.015-0.1 mg/kg/day	
Ca chloride 10%	IV	10-30 mg/kg max: 1 g	q 15-30 minutes
Ca gluconate 10%	IV	100 mg/kg max: 2 g	q 15-30 minutes
Defibrillation		atrial: 0.5 J/kg ventricular: 2 J/kg	double and repeat if unsuccessful
Dextrose 25%	IV	1 ml/kg	check blood sugar
Diazepam	IV	0.1-0.2 mg/kg	as necessary
Epinephrine	IV ET	0.1 ml/kg (1:10,000) 0.1 ml/kg (1:1,000)	q 5-10 minutes
Fentanyl	IV	3-10 µg/kg	q 1-2 hours
Flumazenil	IV	0.2 mg (2 ml) over 30 sec. Repeat using 0.3 mg (3 ml). Further doses 0.5 mg. Max: 5 mg	q 30 seconds
Glucagon	IV	0.025-0.1 mg/kg	q 20-30 minutes
Hydralazine	IV	0.15 mg/kg	q 4-6 hours
Kayexalate	PR	1 g/kg	q 6 hours
Lidocaine	IV	1 mg/kg	q 5-10 minutes
Lorazepam	IV	0.03-0.1 mg/kg max: 4 g	q 15 minutes
Mannitol	IV	0.25-1.0 g/kg	q 2-3 hours
Methohexital	IV	1-2 mg/kg/dose	
Methoxamine	IV	0.1-0.25 mg/kg	q 15 minutes
Metolazone	PO	0.2-0.4 mg/kg/day	divided q 12 hours
Midazolam	IV	0.05-0.2 mg/kg	q 1-2 hours
Morphine	IV	0.1 mg/kg	q 1-2 hours
Naloxone	IV	0.1 mg/kg	q 15-30 minutes
Nifedipine	SL	0.25-0.5 mg/kg	q 6-8 hours
Pancuronium	IV	0.1 mg/kg	q 1 hour
Paraldehyde	Rectal	0.3 ml/kg. max: 5 ml	q 4-6 hours
Pentobarbital	IV	2 mg/kg	q 2-3 hours
Phenobarbital	IV	10-20 mg/kg total loading	3 divided doses over 1-2 hours

Table E-4.   Commonly used emergency drugs (Continued)

Agent	Route	Dose	Frequency
Phenytoin	IV	15 mg/kg total loading	3 divided doses over 1-2 hours **slowly**
Ranitidine	IV	1.0 mg/kg	q 6 hours
Sodium chloride 3%	IV	5 ml/kg (to raise serum Na 4 mEq/L)	once, check serum sodium
Tolazoline	IV	1-2 mg/kg/dose	infusion 1-2 mg/kg/hour
Vecuronium	IV	0.1 mg/kg	q 30-60 minutes
Verapamil	IV	0.1-0.2 mg/kg	may repeat in 30 minutes

Table E-5. Infusions

Drug	Dilution	Concentration	Usual dose range
Amrinone	250 mg in 250 ml	1000 µg/ml	Bolus: 0.75 mg/kg Infusion: 5-10 µg/kg/min
Dobutamine	200 mg in 250 ml 400 mg in 250 ml 800 mg in 250 ml	800 µg/ml 1600 µg/ml 3200 µg/ml	2-10 µg/kg/min
Dopamine	200 mg in 250 ml 400 mg in 250 ml 800 mg in 250 ml	800 µg/ml 1600 µg/ml 3200 µg/ml	2-25 µg/kg/min
Epinephrine	0.25 mg in 250 ml 1.0 mg in 250 ml	1 µg/ml 4 µg/ml	0.02-1 µg/kg/min
Fentanyl	1.0 mg in 50 ml 2.0 mg in 50 ml	20 µg/ml 40 µg/ml	2-10 µg/kg/hr
Heparin	10,000 units in 250 ml	40 units/ml	Bolus: 50 units/kg Infusion: 10-25 units/kg/hr
Isoproterenol	1.0 mg in 100 ml 1.0 mg in 50 ml	10 µg/ml 20 µg/ml	0.05-1 µg/kg/min
Lidocaine	500 mg in 250 ml 1 g in 250 ml 2 g in 250 ml	2000 µg/ml 4000 µg/ml 8000 µg/ml	20 -50 µg/kg/min
Midazolam	12 mg in 50 ml 24 mg in 50 ml	240 µg/ml 480 µg/ml	0.4 -2 µg/kg/min max: 6 µg/kg/min
Nitroprusside	50 mg in 250 ml	200 µg/ml	0.5-10 µg/kg/min
Prostaglandin E_1	0.25 mg in 80 ml	3 µg/ml	0.05-0.1 µg/kg/min
Vasopressin	10 U in 1000 ml	10 milliunits/ml	Esophageal varices: 0.3 U/kg bolus Infusion: 70 milliunits/kg/hr DI: 3 milliunits/kg/hr

Insulin Coverage

Table F-1.   Insulin coverage

Scales for supplemental coverage at 0600, 1130, 1630, 2000, and 0300	
(coverage for ketones and/or increased blood sugar with **regular** insulin)	
Coverage for ketones <u>always</u> overrides coverage for increased sugar	
If blood sugar > 180:	
Small ketones	10% of total daily dose as a supplement
Moderate ketones	15% of total daily dose as a supplement
Large ketones	20% of total daily dose as a supplement
If blood sugar < 180	
Small ketones	5% of total daily dose as a supplement
Moderate ketones	7.5% of total daily dose as a supplement
Large ketones	10% of total daily dose as a supplement

If a patient has ketones in the 6 AM void and has not had any ketones in the last 12 hours of the midnight or 3 AM chemstrip was less than 80, **DO NOT cover for ketones**, but use the coverage based on blood sugar. This elevated sugar and urinary ketones may be a **Somogyi phenomenon**.

Table F-2.   Coverage for blood sugar

At: 6:00 AM, 11:30 AM, 4:30 PM, 8:00 PM				
Chemstrip	10-20 kg	20-40 kg	40-60 kg	60-80 kg
180-240	1 u R	1 u R	2 u R	2 u R
240-320	1 u R	2 u R	3 u R	4 u R
320-400	2 u R	3 u R	4 u R	6 u R
For 12:00 midnight and 3:00 AM				
180-240	---------	---------	2 u R	2 u R
240-320	1 u R	2 u R	2 u R	3 u R
320-400	2 u R	2 u R	3 u R	4 u R

NOTE: 1 U can be added to a basal dose; do not give 1 U as a single separate dose.

Diabetic protocol. Section of Endocrinology, Department of Pediatrics, Children's Hospital of Michigan, Detroit.

Laboratory Findings in Patients with Abnormal Serum Sodium

Table G-1. Laboratory findings in patients with abnormal serum sodium

	Serum			Urine						
	Na (mEq/L)	K (mEq/L)	osm (mOsm/L)	Na (mEq/L)	K (mEq/L)	osm (mOsm/L)	sp. gr	BUN/UUN	FE_{Na} (%)	Urine volume
Hypernatremic dehydration	↑	↔	↑	< 40	↔	> 500	> 1.030	> 1:10	< 1	↓
ATN		variable		> 40	↔	≡ serum	≡ 1.010	< 1:10	> 3	↑ or ↓
SIADH	↓	↔	↓	> 40	↑	> 300	> 1.020	> 1:20	>1 <3	↓
DI	↑	↔	↑	< 10	↓	< 100	< 1.005	< 1:5	< 1	↑
Salt poisoning	↑	↔	↑	> 50	↔	> 300	↔ or ↑	variable	> 3	↔
Factitious hyponatremia* (e.g., hyperglycemia)	↓	↑ or ↓	↑	variable	↑	> 250	↔ or ↑	variable	> 1	↑ or ↔
Pseudohyponatremia (hyperlipidemia)	↓	↔	↔	↔	↔	↔	↔	variable	< 1	↔
Adrenal insufficiency	↓	↑	↓	>40	↓	↔	↔	↔	> 1	variable

*An increase of blood sugar by 100 mg/dL reduces S_{Na} by 1.6 mEq/L because of ECF dilution.

Source: Ashok P. Sarnaik, MD, Chief, Critical Care Medicine, Children's Hospital of Michigan.

Toxicology Panels (Detroit Medical Center/University Laboratories)

Table H-1. Serum drug screen[a]

Acetaminophen	Cocaine (benzoylecgonine)	Alcohols
Salicylates	Opiates	ethanol
Benzodiazepines	Cyclic antidepressants	methanol
Barbiturates	Ethylene glycol (specifically requested)	isopropanol acetone

[a]Send minimum 3 ml whole blood in lavender top tube.

Table H-2. Urine drug screen[a]

Amphetamine	Cocaine (benzoylecgonine)
Barbiturates	Opiates
Benzodiazepines	Phencyclidine
Cannabinoids	Propoxyphene
Methadone	

[a]Send minimum of 50 ml urine.

Comprehensive drug screen

- Serum and urine drug screen panels
- HPLC (REMEDY) screens for approximately 300 drugs and metabolites. Should be used when unknown or uncertain ingestion is strongly suspected.

NOTE: Toxicology panels vary between institutions.

Frequently Used Phone Numbers

Service	Extension	Page number
Admitting		
Allergy/Immunology		
Anesthesiology		
Blood Bank		
Cardiology		
Code Blue		
Emergency Department		
Endocrinology		
ENT		
Gastroenterology		
Genetics		
General Surgery		
Hematology-Oncology		
House Senior/ Chief Resident		
ICU		
Infectious Diseases		
IV Team		
Juvenile Court		

Laboratory
  Microbiology
  Chemistry
  Hematology
  Virology
  Urine		

Medical Records		
NICU		
Nephrology		
Neurology		
Neurosurgery		
Ophthalmology		
Oral Surgery		
Organ Procurement		

Service	Extension	Page number
Orthopedics		
Pathology		
Pharmacology/Toxicology		
Poison Control		
Pulmonary		

Radiology
   CT Scan
   Interventional
   File Room
   Dictated Reports		

Respiratory Therapy		
Security		
Social Service/Child Protection Team		
State Screen		
Transport Team		
Urology		

Suggested Readings

AIDS Etiology, Diagnosis, Treatment and Prevention, 1992, 3rd ed. Devita VT, et al. Lippincott.

The Battered Child, 1987. Helfer RE, Kempe RS. University of Chicago Press.

Clinical Management of Poisoning and Drug Overdose, 1990, 2nd ed. Haddad LM. Saunders.

Critical Care Clinics, vol 3 no 3, July 1987: Acute Spinal Cord Injury. Albin MS. Saunders.

Critical Care Clinics, vol 1, no 1, March 1985: Burns. Wachtel TL. Saunders.

Critical Care Clinics, vol 9, no 2, April 1993: Circulatory Shock. Rackow EC, Astiz ME. Saunders.

DeGowin and DeGowin's Bedside Diagnostic Examination, 1981, 4th ed. DeGowin RL. Macmillan.

Diagnosis of Stupor and Coma, 1982. Plum F, Posner JB. F. A. Davis.

Diagnostic Imaging of Child Abuse, 1987. Kleinman P (ed). Williams & Wilkins.

Emergency Medicine Clinics of North America, vol 9, no 3, August 1991: Pediatric Emergencies. Burkle FM, Wiebe RA. Saunders.

Emergency Medicine, Concepts and Clinical Practice, 1992. Rosen P, Barkin RM. Mosby-Year Book.

Emergency Pediatrics: A Guide to Ambulatory Care, 1990, 3rd ed. Barkin RM, Rosen P. Mosby.

Essentials of Pediatric Intensive Care, 1990. Levin DL, Morriss FC. Quality Medical Publishing.

Essentials of Pediatric Intensive Care Manual, 1992. Toro-Figueroa LO. Quality Medical Publishing.

Gellis & Kagan's Current Pediatric Therapy, 1993. Burg F. Saunders.

Goldfrank's Toxicologic Emergencies, 1994, 5th ed. Goldfrank LR, et al. Appleton & Lange.

Goodman and Gilman's The Pharmacological Basis of Therapeutics, 1990, 8th ed. Goodman Gilman A. Pergamon Press.

Hematology for Infancy and Childhood, 1993, 4th ed. Nathan DG, Oski FA. Saunders.

Hematology/Oncology Clinics of North America, vol 6, no 5, October 1992: Coagulation Disorders I. Saunders.

Infectious Diseases of Children, 1992, 9th ed. Krugman S. Mosby-Year Book.

The Management of Trauma. 1985, 4th ed. Zuidema GD, et al. Saunders.

Medical Toxicology, Diagnosis and Treatment of Human Poisoning, 1988. Ellenhorn MJ, Barceloux DG. Elsevier.

Micromedex Computerized Clinical Information System: Poisindex.

National Asthma Education Program, Expert Panel Report, Executive Summary, 1991. Guidelines for the Diagnosis and Management of Asthma. U. S. Department of Health and Human Services.

Nelson Textbook of Pediatrics, 1992, 14th ed. Behrman RE. Saunders.

Pediatric Cardiology for Practitioners, 1988, 2nd ed. Park MK. Year Book.

Pediatric Clinics of North America vol 39, no 5, October 1992: Child Abuse Intervention in the Emergency Room. Hyden PW, Gallagher TA. Saunders.

Pediatric Clinics of North America, vol 40, no 2, April 1993: Transporting the Neurologically Compromised Child: Sarnaik AP, Lieh-Lai MW. In Transport Medicine: Jaimovich DB, Vidyasagar D. Saunders.

Pediatric Emergency Medicine, 1993, 1st ed. Reisdorff EJ, Roberts MR, Wiegenstein JG. Saunders.

Pediatric Emergency Medicine, Concepts and Clinical Practice, 1992. Barkin RM. Mosby-Year Book.

Pediatric Neurology for the House Officer, 1988, 3rd ed. Weiner HL. Williams & Wilkins.

Pediatric Textbook of Fluids and Electrolytes, 1990. Ichikawa I. Williams & Wilkins.

Pediatrics in Review, vol 12, no 9, March 1991. Lusher JM, Warrier I: Hemophilia. American Academy of Pediatrics.

Pediatrics in Review, vol 14, no 5, May 1993. Jung FF, Ingelfinger JR: Hypertension in Childhood and Adolescence. American Academy of Pediatrics.

Principles and Practice of Pediatric Oncology, 1993, 2nd ed. Pizzo PA, Poplack DG. Lippincott.

Principles and Practice of Pediatrics, 1994, 2nd ed. Oski FA. Lippincott.

The Red Book: Report of the Committee on Infectious Diseases, 1994. American Academy of Pediatrics.

Rudolph's Pediatrics, 1991, 19th ed. Rudolph AM. Appleton & Lange.

Textbook of Pediatric Advanced Life Support, 1990. Chameides L. American Heart Association.

Textbook of Pediatric Emergency Medicine, 1993, 3rd ed. Fleischer GR, Ludwig S. Williams & Wilkins.

Textbook of Pediatric Infectious Diseases, 1992, 3rd ed. Feigin RD, Cherry JD. Saunders.

Textbook of Pediatric Intensive Care, 1992, 2nd ed. Rogers MC. Williams & Wilkins.

Water and Electrolytes in Pediatrics: Physiology, Pathology, and Treatment, 1993, 2nd ed. Finberg L. Saunders.

Williams Textbook of Endocrinology, 1985, 7th ed. Wilson JD, Foster DF. Saunders.

Wintrobe's Clinical Hematology, 1993, 9th ed. Lee GR, et al. Lea & Febiger.

Notes

Index